Palgrave Studies in Literature, Science and Medicine

Series Editors
Sharon Ruston
Dept. of English and Creative Writing
Lancaster University, Lancaster, United Kingdom

Alice Jenkins
School of Critical Studies
University of Glasgow, Glasgow, United Kingdom

Catherine Belling
Feinberg School of Medicine, Northwestern University
Chicago, Illinois, USA

Palgrave Studies in Literature, Science and Medicine is an exciting new series that focuses on one of the most vibrant and interdisciplinary areas in literary studies: the intersection of literature, science and medicine. Comprised of academic monographs, essay collections, and Palgrave Pivot books, the series will emphasize a historical approach to its subjects, in conjunction with a range of other theoretical approaches. The series will cover all aspects of this rich and varied field and is open to new and emerging topics as well as established ones.

Editorial board: Steven Connor, Professor of English, University of Cambridge, UK; Lisa Diedrich, Associate Professor in Women's and Gender Studies, Stony Brook University, USA; Kate Hayles, Professor of English, Duke University, USA; Peter Middleton, Professor of English, University of Southampton, UK; Sally Shuttleworth, Professorial Fellow in English, St Anne's College, University of Oxford, UK; Susan Squier, Professor of Women's Studies and English, Pennsylvania State University, USA; Martin Willis, Professor of English, University of Westminster, UK.

More information about this series at
http://www.springer.com/series/14613

Martina Zimmermann

The Poetics and Politics of Alzheimer's Disease Life-Writing

palgrave
macmillan

Martina Zimmermann
King's College, London
London, United Kingdom

Palgrave Studies in Literature, Science and Medicine
ISBN 978-3-319-44387-4   ISBN 978-3-319-44388-1 (eBook)
DOI 10.1007/978-3-319-44388-1

Library of Congress Control Number: 2016952436

© The Editor(s) (if applicable) and The Author(s) 2017. This book is an open access publication.
Open Access This book is licensed under the terms of the Creative Commons Attribution 4.0 International License (http://creativecommons.org/licenses/by/4.0/), which permits use, sharing, adaptation, distribution and reproduction in any medium or format, as long as you give appropriate credit to the original author(s) and the source, provide a link to the Creative Commons license and indicate if changes were made.
The images or other third party material in this book are included in the book's Creative Commons license, unless indicated otherwise in a credit line to the material. If material is not included in the book's Creative Commons license and your intended use is not permitted by statutory regulation or exceeds the permitted use, you will need to obtain permission directly from the copyright holder.
The use of general descriptive names, registered names, trademarks, service marks, etc. in this publication does not imply, even in the absence of a specific statement, that such names are exempt from the relevant protective laws and regulations and therefore free for general use.
The publisher, the authors and the editors are safe to assume that the advice and information in this book are believed to be true and accurate at the date of publication. Neither the publisher nor the authors or the editors give a warranty, express or implied, with respect to the material contained herein or for any errors or omissions that may have been made. The publisher remains neutral with regard to jurisdictional claims in published maps and institutional affiliations.

Cover pattern © Melisa Hasan

Printed on acid-free paper

This Palgrave Macmillan imprint is published by Springer Nature
The registered company is Springer International Publishing AG
The registered company address is: Gewerbestrasse 11, 6330 Cham, Switzerland

Acknowledgements

The template for this volume was laid down during my study towards an MA in Literature and Medicine at King's College London. The participation in this course was generously supported by the Lesmüller Foundation, Germany. The research underpinning the reworking and expanding of my MA dissertation with a view to publication has been undertaken with generous funding from the Wellcome Trust [099351/Z/12/Z], which also enables open access publication of this book.

I am sincerely grateful to Brian Hurwitz, Neil Vickers and James Whitehead. Brian's and Neil's enthusiasm and curiosity in welcoming me to their MA programme carried me a long way on a steep learning curve and the course's formidable reading list. I am particularly thankful to Brian, who was my personal tutor throughout the course: he tirelessly challenged my claims, and set the bar high for what could pass as truly interdisciplinary writing. To Neil, I owe thanks for insightful discussion on illness life-writing as well as psychoanalytical perspectives on the dementia experience; and to Jamie, I am indebted for deepening my comprehension of concepts such as closure and narrative truth. All three offered invaluable criticism and helpful comments on drafts of this manuscript. Their variously differing perspectives on the Health Humanities have significantly shaped my own thinking about interdisciplinarity, and are inspiration to persevere at the boundary between the Sciences and the Humanities.

I began active research in the Health Humanities during full-time employment in a Science department, and could not have embarked on this work without approval from my Science mentor Jochen Klein. As his open-mindedness has given me the space to try out new teaching approaches, his magnanimous nature granted me the time to enrol on this course. Only in the awareness of his quiet confidence that I would be able to follow my academic duties and research activities, while simultaneously seizing this opportunity, could I find the mental space to dedicate myself to this experience. I could not have hoped or wished for more support.

I also thank Susan Greenfield and Martin Westwell for their backing and encouragement in applying for the MA programme at King's.

Throughout working on this book, I had the opportunity to teach illness narratives in a Pharmaceutical/Medical Sciences as well as a Health Humanities context. The experience of practical and conceptual disciplinary limits and limitations confirms my believe that the Health Humanities must eventually complement the Sciences from within; that only a firm scientific grounding will enable an appreciation of the Health Humanities that is removed from discourses of usefulness. I am indebted to all undergraduate students who entered into exploring a field outside textbook physiology and pharmacology, both in the Pharmaceutical Sciences Department at Goethe University Frankfurt and at the School of Biomedical Sciences at King's. Teaching at graduate level in the English Department at King's, and discussing my research in several postgraduate seminars in Frankfurt enormously enriched my understanding of what the Sciences and Humanities each take for granted – in terms of methodology as much as terminology.

In my *Antrittsvorlesung* as *Privatdozentin*, I had occasion finally to present to my Science colleagues the interdisciplinary teaching approaches in Pharmaceutical Care that had paralleled my scientific research in Frankfurt. Among those attending, I particularly wish to thank Jennifer Dressman, Gunter Eckert, Michael Karas, Paul Layer, Rolf Marschalek, Martin Pos and Thomas Prisner for their interest and observations.

I also presented some of my research and teaching ideas at a range of Health Humanities meetings. The comments of many have refined and further motivated this work; I specifically want to mention Jens Brockmeier, Michael Clark, Peter Frommelt, Eileen Gillooly, Brian Glasser, Nortin Hadler, Terry Holt, Hannah Landecker, Tom Linden, Gordon McMullan, Maria Medved, Columba Quigley, Barry Saunders, David Stone and Jane Thrailkill.

I also extend my gratitude to the anonymous reader for the constructive and perceptive consideration of my work; to Ben Doyle for editorial support at Palgrave; and to those who believed in this research long before it had taken shape as this book: Carolin Duttlinger, Joe Harris, Peter Howarth and, most of all, Steven Brown.

Contents

1 **Introduction** 1
   Alzheimer's Disease and Narrative Theory: Is 'Narrating Dementia' an Oxymoron? 7
   Conscientious Criticism: Mapping My Reading of Dementia Life-Writing 12
   Sifting Dementia Narratives 19

2 **Of Wives and Daughters: Stereotypes of the Caring Female?** 23
   The Lost Identity: Alzheimer's Disease, Adult Children and the Past 27
   Times Are Changing: 'Mothers' and Lovers 33
   Perceived Caregiver Burden and Patient Identity Condition Each Other 40

3 **From a 'Care-Free' Distance: Sons Talking About Cultural Concepts** 49
   Body and Mind: The Patient as Object 53
   Alzheimer's and Aging: The Patient as Subject 62
   Historical, Cultural and Personal Context Influence Attitudes to Dementia 68

4 About Tradition and Triumph: Patients Popularise
   Dementia Narrative   75
   Tradition Sells: The Journey into Darkness   78
   *Form and Contents: Narrating Alzheimer's versus
   'Account-Ability'*   83
   *Collaborative Writing Meets Societal Norms and Political
   Intentions*   91

5 On Reclaiming Authority: The Enabling Discourse of
   Alzheimer's Disease   95
   Times Are Changing II: Patient Activism   98
   Identity within Dementia: The Patient as Postmodern Prophet? 103
   The Patient's World Advises Caregiver and Society   110

6 Conclusion   117
   *Alzheimer's Disease Narratives Today: New Media,
   Germane Stories*   119
   Stories of Dementia: Pedagogical, Political, Representative 128

Bibliography of Dementia Narratives   133

Works Cited   141

Index   157

CHAPTER 1

Introduction

Critically Reading Dementia Narratives: Amplifying Advocacy

Abstract The introduction gives an overview on sociopolitical and research-related developments regarding dementia, and attempts explanations for why the interest in dementia of critical scholarship continues to be very limited and particularly focused on caregiver accounts. It illustrates that an understanding of the obvious neglect of dementia patient narratives sheds some light onto the ethical implications and challenges of critically reading such narratives: these narratives seem least of all fit to match classical survivor illness literature, and serious impairment in the ability to tell or understand stories has been taken as motivation to neglect patient narratives. Approaches highlighting the importance of pre-narrative identity and a growing body of psycho-philosophical work demand a closer scrutiny of patient narratives, which would also amplify their author-narrators' advocacy.

Keywords Advocacy · Book market · Demography · Dysnarrativia · Narrative identity

> Anyone who has experienced living with this disease as a caregiver or as one who has the disease knows that its effects are devastating. Lives are turned upside down, long-held plans for the future become wistful musings over what might have been, the long-anticipated 'golden years' become tarnished with pain, sadness, and irreversible, inexorable loss.[1]
>
> Understanding how Alzheimer's is perceived and represented can help interrupt and change the experience of the disease for those who suffer, those who anticipate suffering, and those who care for its victims.[2]

As a scientist, I have worked in laboratories where studies are carried out to identify whether individual molecular parameters within specific cells are correlated with the progression of neurodegenerative processes in conditions like Alzheimer's disease. On one occasion, while blood was being drawn from a patient, I chatted with the elderly lady, who all the while showed herself happily aware of being involved in a research project. I remember an animated exchange, laughter, stories from the past. Later that day, I met her again as she was pushed along the aisle of the outpatient department in a wheelchair. I waved at her, but she looked straight through me. I alluded to our earlier conversation, but she peered at me blankly, asking me for my name. I felt perplexed and I had no idea how to react. A nurse's call from a nearby examination room ended this encounter.

On my way back home I felt disturbed: how could I have reacted like this? It was as if I had not even considered that the subjects included in such studies, if they were not healthy controls, had a diagnosis like 'probable Alzheimer's'. It was as if I had not been aware of the implications of 'short-term memory problems'. I was researching in the lab all day, but what did I really know about Alzheimer's disease? I was working on molecular mechanisms underlying the pathogenesis of Alzheimer's disease. But I had no clue what it was like to encounter, and engage with a patient. I had textbook knowledge and gathered facts from specialised journals. But I had no grasp of how the condition was lived with in daily life. I was exposed to what might be called the cultural mainstream Alzheimer's narrative that feeds – originating from a medico-scientific dementia discourse – on popular scientific texts and mass media coverage. Indeed, given their intense

---

[1] Steven R. Sabat, *The Experience of Alzheimer's Disease. Life through a Tangled Veil* (Oxford: Blackwell Publishers Ltd., 2001), p. vii (Sabat 2001).

[2] Anne Davis Basting, 'Looking back from loss: views of the self in Alzheimer's disease', *Journal of Aging Studies*, 17 (2003), pp. 87–99, p. 88 (Basting 2003).

and continued contact with mainstream-moulding medico-scientific concepts and images, researchers are perhaps even more directly exposed to this mainstream narrative than any other lay person; the term lay person including all those who have not lived the experience of being in the presence of someone with the condition. But what does this mainstream narrative tell? What realities define how the mainstream thinks about Alzheimer's? And how does all this relate to my encounter?

Alzheimer's disease is the most common neurodegenerative disorder among the elderly. In view of major demographic changes, it has reached epidemic proportions in the developed world during the last thirty years. More than twenty-six million people suffer worldwide – 1.5 percent of the American population, 1.2 percent of the UK population, and by the year 2050 this number is expected to triple. The condition presents as an early as well as the more well-known late-onset form. Patients afflicted by the early-onset form are as young as forty-five when they are diagnosed, and account for approximately two percent of Alzheimer's patients. Late-onset Alzheimer's disease, in turn, is defined as afflicting individuals aged sixty-five years or older. Patients face memory loss, an impaired ability to understand or produce speech and an inability to recognise things or people. Most of all, they are aware that their mental acuity continually declines, and their perception of themselves as individual persons disappears in a relentless process of brain atrophy.[3] Regardless of their age of onset, patients usually have five to ten years between diagnosis and death. During this period, they pass through different stages of the condition, with early stages still allowing for the patient's articulation. Later stages strongly limit intellectual performance, making the patient dependent on caregiving in almost all activities of daily life. Drugs are currently only of limited symptomatic effect.

In the light of such numbers and such constant – and increasing – presence, Alzheimer's disease has come to embody fears of illness, aging and death.[4] It meanwhile represents dementia itself; not the neuroscientific

---

[3] Ove Almkvist, 'Neuropsychological features of early Alzheimer's disease: preclinical and clinical stages', *Acta Neurologica Scandinavica Supplementum*, 165 (1996), pp. 63–71 (Almkvist 1996).

[4] Norm O'Rourke, 'Alzheimer's disease as a metaphor for contemporary fears of aging', *Journal of the American Geriatrics Society*, 44 (1996), pp. 220–221 (O'Rourke 1996).

description of a specific pathology that is defined in terms of the degeneration and death of specific populations of nerve cells in the hippocampal and cortical areas of the brain.[5] In direct consequence, the condition no longer stands only for the individual's profound cognitive decline, increasing behavioural difficulties and substantive memory erosion. It has become a term heavily loaded with stigma, as the cultural mainstream narrative of Alzheimer's disease centres on fears of caregiver burden, dependence, passivity and vulnerability.[6]

Throughout the 1970s and 1980s, research into Alzheimer's disease was essentially exclusively the domain of the biomedical sciences. Only following several political decisions during this period, did Alzheimer's disease begin to gain public attention. In 1974, the National Institute on Aging (NIA) was founded in the United States, making 'problems and diseases of the aged' the centre of its funding interest. The NIA's efforts regarding the dissemination of health information carried Alzheimer's disease into research laboratories as well as increasing public awareness; the creation of the Alzheimer Disease and Related Disorders Association (today the Alzheimer's Association) in 1979 and Alzheimer's Disease International (ADI) in 1984, initiated by Australia, Canada, the United States and the United Kingdom, had a similar effect. Further European countries joined in 1986 and 1987, among them France, Germany and Italy; Spain and Austria followed in 1993 and 1994, respectively.[7]

These sociopolitical and research-related developments led to a quickly rising media attention and interest in dementia. Additionally, an ever increasing number of narratives relating the illness experience provided testimony to the hardship in the confrontation with incremental, chronic and untreatable cognitive decline. The early 1990s brought the patient's first-person narrative

---

[5] John H. Morrison and Patrick R. Hof, 'Selective vulnerability of corticocortical and hippocampal circuits in aging and Alzheimer's disease', *Progress in Brain Research*, 136 (2002), pp. 467–486 (Morrison and Hof 2002).

[6] See, for example, Hannah Zeilig, 'Dementia as a cultural metaphor', *The Gerontologist*, 54 (2014), pp. 258–267 (Zeilig 2014); Martina Zimmermann, 'Alzheimer's disease metaphors as mirror and lens to the stigma of dementia', *Literature and Medicine* (forthcoming Spring 2017) (Zimmermann forthcoming).

[7] For a short account of the medico-scientific history of Alzheimer's disease, see, e.g., François Boller, 'History of dementia', *Handbook of Clinical Neurology*, 89 (2008), pp. 3–13 (Boller 2008); Stanley Finger, 'The neuropathology of memory', in *Origins of Neuroscience* (New York: Oxford University Press, 1994), pp. 349–368 (Finger 1994).

to the attention of a wider audience. J. Bernlef's *Out of Mind* appeared in 1988 as the first book-length fictional account consistently told from the patient's point of view.[8] Robert Davis's *My Journey into Alzheimer's Disease* was its first book-length Alzheimer's patient autobiographical counterpart.[9] Subsequently, in 1993, Diana Friel McGowin's *Living in the Labyrinth* attracted international attention to dementia patient accounts.[10] Other publications have followed, though the number of dementia patients voicing their experiences in book-length narratives still barely rises above a dozen. Similarly, the surge of Alzheimer's disease caregiver narratives commenced only eighteen years ago, when John Bayley's *Iris Trilogy* provoked international resonance – certainly enhanced by Richard Eyre's 2001 movie adaptation.[11] That the Wellcome Trust Book Prize has been awarded to an Alzheimer's caregiver narrative in 2009, and only two years later to a fictional story featuring the condition, signals continued sociocultural concern with the condition.[12]

But the encounter with the elderly lady confronted me with questions whose consideration appeared to be absent from this mainstream narrative, namely, how do patients and caregivers cope with dementia in daily life; how do they experience memory loss; and, above all, how do they negotiate with this very narrative. For this reason I began reading Alzheimer's disease-related accounts, both fiction and life-writing. These narratives put into perspective my research, for example, with sterile cell culture models. With each narrative I felt the tension between fact and fiction increase. The questions I increasingly asked could less and less be answered by the research I was pursuing; and the ways in which patients in particular told about their

---

[8] J. Bernlef [pseud. of Hendrik Jan Marsman], *Out of Mind* (London: Faber and Faber, 1988) (Bernlef 1988); the Dutch original *Hersenschimmen* was published in 1984. Contemporary critical reception linked the protagonist's experience to Alzheimer's disease; see: Anita Desai, 'The narrator has Alzheimer's', *New York Times*, 17 September 1989 (Desai 1989).

[9] Robert Davis, *My Journey into Alzheimer's Disease. Helpful Insights for Family and Friends. A True Story* (Carol Stream: Tyndale House Publishers, 1989) (Davis 1989).

[10] Diana Friel McGowin, *Living in the Labyrinth. A Personal Journey through the Maze of Alzheimer's* (New York: Dell Publishing, 1993) (McGowin 1993).

[11] John Bayley, *The Iris Trilogy* (London: Abacus, 2003) (Bayley 2003); all references from this edition are incorporated in the text; *Iris: A Memoir of Iris Murdoch* was originally published in 1998; Richard Eyre, *Iris* (BBC, 2001) (Eyre 2001).

[12] Andrea Gillies, *Keeper. Living with Nancy. A Journey into Alzheimer's* (London: Short Books, 2009) (Gillies 2009); Alice LaPlante, *Turn of Mind* (London: Harvill Secker, 2011) (LaPlante 2011).

illness experience related only partly to the medico-scientific evidence as I studied it, and matched the mainstream narrative very little. Wanting to immerse myself more deeply in these texts, I however noticed how comparatively small the critical scholarship focusing on dementia narrative was. Symptomatic of this phenomenon, Jeffrey Aronson classified Bayley's memoir as 'bereavement' literature in the year 2000, instead of introducing a category like 'dementia', and has yet to revise his classification over a decade later.[13] Also, work on discourse analysis lamented, as recently as 2014, that 'little research has addressed how people with the condition and their caregivers speak or write of the condition themselves'.[14]

This observation underscores my own conviction that dementia narrative continues to be undervalued as a separate body of specific illness lifewriting. In view of current major demographic changes, I consider Alzheimer's disease *the* illness of stigma and fear. Succumbing or not to memory loss and the threatening consequences highlighted by Steven R. Sabat, Western society is rapidly aging and, as such, will be increasingly confronted with age-related forms of dementia and its identity-threatening consequences on a daily basis. My literary analysis here of dementia narratives attends to the imbalance between the sociocultural and medico-scientific preoccupation with Alzheimer's disease, on the one hand, and the obvious invisibility of the individuals directly concerned in both humanities scholarship and current policy discussions, on the other hand. In particular, it aims at amplifying the voice and advocacy of patients and caregivers, and critically appraising the poetics and politics of their telling. This approach will complement what Nicole Müller and Robert W. Schrauf term '[t]he

---

[13] Jeffrey Aronson, 'Autopathography: the patient's tale', *Biomedical Journal*, 321 (2000), pp. 1599–1602 (Aronson 2000), and http://www.clinpharm.ox.ac.uk/JKA/patientstale; I had accessed this page in March 2011; following a University of Oxford website reorganisation, I was not able to access this page from September 2013 onwards. Aronson's newly created page, 'The patients' tales collection', https://sites.google.com/a/patientstales.org/home/home (accessed August 2016), wonderfully collects examples from the whole range of illness auto-pathographies; that this site does not list dementia patient narratives further testifies to the minimal number of texts as well as the lacking general awareness of their existence.

[14] Vaidehi Ramanathan, 'Alzheimer pathographies. Glimpses into how people with AD and their caregivers text themselves', in *Dialogue and Dementia. Cognitive and Communicative Resources for Engagement*, ed. by Robert W. Schrauf and Nicole Müller (New York: Psychology Press, 2014), pp. 245–261, p. 245 (Ramanathan 2014).

atomistic, dissociation-focused view of cognitive and linguistic impairment', whose consequences my own story illustrates.[15] And it will, as Anne Davis Basting suggests, further a necessary understanding of the patient's and caregiver's perception of cognitive impairment.

Such an understanding begins with a search for potential explanations for why the literary scholarship concerned with Alzheimer's disease narratives continues to be very limited and particularly focused on caregiver accounts. Indeed, initially I want to understand how the obvious neglect of dementia patient narratives sheds some light onto the ethical implications and challenges of critiquing such narratives.

Alzheimer's Disease and Narrative Theory: Is 'Narrating Dementia' an Oxymoron?

In her work on *Illness and the Limits of Expression*, Kathlyn Conway is particularly concerned with the fact that American culture strongly thrives on the idea that 'anything is possible'. It is weary, she submits, of placing illness per se as well as writing about it into the centre of public scrutiny, since:

> The emphasis on youth, physical strength, and beauty not only constitutes a denial of illness and dying but also causes illness to be viewed as anomalous and relegated to the separate world of medicine.

Considering the prognosis of Alzheimer's disease – that is, its very degenerative chronicity – a narrative of dementia does seem least of all fit to match classical survivor illness literature. Conway explicitly investigates less popular, since non-triumphalist, types of illness narrative that place particular emphasis on otherness through illness. Her critical analysis enhances the reader's appreciation of the complex relationship between body and mind, and draws particular attention to literature that 'looks more squarely at the devastating reality of serious illness or disability'.[16]

---

[15] Nicole Müller and Robert W. Schrauf, 'Conversation as cognition. Reframing cognition in dementia', in *Dialogue and Dementia*, ed. by Schrauf and Müller, pp. 3–26, p. 3 (Müller and Schrauf 2014).

[16] Kathlyn Conway, *Illness and the Limits of Expression* (Ann Arbor: The University of Michigan Press, 2007), pp. 6, 4, 8 (Conway 2007); also note Lisa Diedrich's deliberations on the American 'improved self' as compared to the British 'ironic self' in much illness life-writing; see: *Treatments. Language, Politics, and the Culture of Illness* (Minneapolis: University of Minnesota Press, 2007), esp. Chap. 3 (Diedrich 2007).

In this context, Conway mentions Arthur W. Frank's conceptualisation of the 'chaos narrative' that mirrors how 'the storyteller experiences life: without sequence or discernible causality'. Frank himself claims that the '[l]ived chaos makes reflection, and consequently storytelling, impossible'. Citing the account of an Alzheimer's disease caregiver, he states that 'the story has no narrative sequence, only an incessant present with no memorable past and no future worth anticipating'.[17] As I read Frank's statement, it lacks a clear distinction between patient and caregiver account and overlooks book-length, coherently told caregiver stories. While I agree that temporal coherence is frequently lacking in patient-authored texts, I still believe their emphasis on significance makes these stories worth telling, reading and pondering.

In his *Stories of Sickness*, Howard Brody goes even further. He recognises that 'having a mind that functions in a fairly normal way is a very important part of being a person', but, in advanced dementia, he continues, 'there is a common-sense aspect to the assertion that the individual "no longer exists as a person"'.[18] This statement is in line with approaches that locate personhood in memory, suggesting that identity is lost in Alzheimer's disease, and subjectivity is altered.[19] Regrettably, Brody does not provide an analysis of patient accounts, which in itself underlines that he sees identity in dementia as being impaired.[20] His view gains additional support from Paul John Eakin's work. Eakin deliberates on the importance of storytelling for the creation of identity, and particularly expands on how serious impairment in the ability to tell or understand

---

[17] Arthur W. Frank, *The Wounded Storyteller. Body, Illness, and Ethics* (Chicago: The University of Chicago Press, 1995), pp. 97, 98, 99 (Frank 1995); Frank specifically expands on the 'chaos narrative' in Chap. 5.

[18] Howard Brody, *Stories of Sickness, 2nd edition* (New York: Oxford University Press, 2003), pp. 67, 69 (Brody 2003).

[19] Pierre-Marie Charazac, 'Loss of identity in Alzheimer's disease: a psychoanalytic approach', *Psychologie et Neuropsychiatrie du Vieillissement*, 7.3 (2009), pp. 169–174 (Charazac 2009); for a critical reflection on the patient's perceived loss of self, see: Elizabeth Herskovits, 'Struggling over subjectivity: debates about the "self" and Alzheimer's disease', *Medical Anthropology Quarterly*, 9.2 (1995), pp. 146–164 (Herskovits 1995).

[20] Where Brody explores ethical issues concerning end-of-life decisions in Alzheimer's disease, he reflects on the patient 'Margo' in the third person; see: *Stories of Sickness*, pp. 247–253 (Brody 2003).

stories severely impacts on our sense of self.[21] Similarly, and in reliance on Eakin, Jerome Bruner affirms that 'the construction of selfhood, it seems, cannot proceed without a capacity to narrate'.[22]

All three authors refer to dementia and Alzheimer's disease as examples of dysnarrativia at a time when several patient-authored dementia narratives had already been published such that these narratives might have accentuated their investigations differently. What is more, recent work on 'narrative scaffolding in dementia' suggests that the act of joint storytelling about shared experiences enables patients to maintain their individual identity. In fact, for Lars-Christer Hydén, 'telling temporally discontinuous narratives does not appear to affect or disrupt the teller's experience of some sort of continuous sense of self and identity'; rather it affects the person without diagnosis, that is, the caregiver.[23] More linguistically focused studies, in turn, highlight the importance of pre-narrative identity for both patient and caregiver.[24]

In line with these affirmations, Jane Crisp's discussion of narratives produced by her cognitively impaired mother is as refreshing as it is reassuring: in introducing external information that serves to elucidate the relevance of specific events in her mother's accounts, Crisp demonstrates that narratives of Alzheimer's patients do not only comply with the norms of narrative, but are functional as means for interaction and recon-

---

[21] Paul John Eakin, *How Our Lives Become Stories. Making Selves* (Ithaca: Cornell University Press, 1999), esp. p. 46 (Eakin 1999) (see below p. 54); on self-narration and identity, see also: Paul John Eakin, *Living Autobiographically. How We Create Identity in Narrative* (Ithaca: Cornell University Press, 2008), esp. pp. 45–59 (Eakin 2008).

[22] Jerome Bruner, *Making Stories. Law, Literature, Life* (Cambridge: Harvard University Press, 2002), p. 86 (Bruner 2002).

[23] Lars-Christer Hydén and L. Örulv, 'Narrative and identity in Alzheimer's disease: a case study', *Journal of Aging Studies*, 23 (2009), pp. 205–214, p. 213 (Hydén and Örulv 2009); see also: Lars-Christer Hydén, 'Narrative collaboration and scaffolding in dementia', *Journal of Aging Studies*, 25 (2011), pp. 339–347 (Hydén 2011).

[24] See, e.g., Vai Ramanathan, *Alzheimer Discourse. Some Sociolinguistic Dimensions* (Mahwah: Lawrence Erlbaum Associates, 1997) (Ramanathan 1997); Julie Goyder, *We'll Be Married in Fremantle* (Fremantle: Fremantle Arts Centre Press, 2001) (Goyder 2001); and, recently, Jens Brockmeier, 'Questions of meaning: memory, dementia, and the post-autobiographical perspective', in *Beyond Loss: Dementia, Identity, Personhood*, ed. by Lars-Christer Hydén, Hilde Lindemann and Jens Brockmeier (New York: Oxford University Press, 2014), pp. 69–90 (Brockmeier 2014).

structing identity.[25] In the same vein, recent narrative-based anthropological studies support the notion of coherence in narratives by dementia patients, even in the absence of factuality.[26] In addition, neuropsychological and social constructionist perspectives have begun focusing on the analysis of the patient's embodied portrayal of their condition; psychoanalytical approaches seek to explain anxieties and mental disturbances in old age with unresolved early psychological constellations; and anthropological fieldwork concentrates on the analysis of caregiver narratives with the aim being to reconstruct the patient's and the caregiver's inner world.[27]

These insights and approaches reinforce work that explores the nature of personal identity in dementia through the prism of psychiatry and philosophy. This research importantly claims that patients:

> should be treated as wholes, with attention not only to their biology, but also to their psychology, their social and ethical concerns, and the cultural and spiritual aspects of their lives.

In particularly analysing patient narratives, Julian C. Hughes and colleagues come to see patients – even those, who are afflicted by moderate to severe stages of dementia – as able to maintain their feelings of self-worth. Specifically, they profess that:

---

[25] Jane Crisp, 'Making sense of the stories that people with Alzheimer's tell: a journey with my mother', *Nursing Inquiry*, 2.3 (1995), pp. 133–140 (Crisp 1995).

[26] Athena Helen McLean, 'Coherence without facticity in dementia: the case of Mrs. Fine', in *Thinking about Dementia: Culture, Loss, and the Anthropology of Senility*, ed. by Annette Leibing and Lawrence Cohen (New Brunswick: Rutgers University Press, 2006), pp. 157–179 (McLean 2006).

[27] Sabat, *The Experience of Alzheimer's Disease* (Sabat 2001); Jaber Gubrium, 'Narrative practice and the inner worlds of the Alzheimer disease experience', in *Concepts of Alzheimer Disease. Biological, Clinical, and Cultural Perspectives*, ed. by Peter J. Whitehouse, Konrad Maurer and Jesse F. Ballenger (Baltimore: The Johns Hopkins University Press, 2000), pp. 181–203 (Gubrium 2000); Margot Waddell, 'Only connect: developmental issues from early to late life', *Psychoanalytic Psychotherapy*, 14 (2000), pp. 239–252 (Waddell 2000); W. Ladson Hinton and Sue Levkoff, 'Constructing Alzheimer's: narratives of lost identities, confusion and loneliness in old age', *Culture, Medicine and Psychiatry*, 23.4 (1999), pp. 453–475 (Hinton and Levkoff 1999).

we need to see the person as a situated human being, who engages with the world in a mental and bodily way in agent-like activities, showing (amongst other things) desires, choices, drives, emotions, needs, and attachments.[28]

This psycho-philosophical body of evidence criticises the biomedical approach as likely reducing and devaluing the individual it has set out to describe.[29] Therefore, a dedicated consideration of the patient's own as compared to the caregiver's word and world is necessary, and, in the awareness of the steadily growing number of autobiographical book-length Alzheimer's disease narratives, most timely. Continuing to neglect patient stories would seem unethical in view of the significant effort patients go to, despite – and since – they are facing their cognitive decline in every sentence they write.

The earliest piece of criticism exclusively focusing on book-published patient narratives (Davis's and McGowin's accounts as well as Cary Smith Henderson's *Partial View*) aimed at understanding how specific texts 'worry over and create a sense of selfhood in the midst of its perceived loss' in the crisis of Alzheimer's disease. While not addressing patient accounts as literary texts, Anne Davis Basting observes how, especially in early patient-authored texts, the language is 'cleansed of the disease', and how narrative form contradicts disease experience. My reading of patient narratives builds on the artist's analysis of how narrative construction serves as an indicator of disease 'performance' or 'description', because it will support a more comprehensive understanding of patients' poetic choices as being politically driven.[30] This is especially true, since Basting's work formed part of the background of important gerontological research by Ellen Bouchard Ryan and colleagues on the 'lived

---

[28] Julian C. Hughes, Stephen J. Louw and Steven R. Sabat, 'Seeing whole', in *Dementia. Mind, Meaning, and the Person*, ed. by Julian C. Hughes, Stephen J. Louw and Steven R. Sabat (New York: Oxford University Press, 2006), pp. 1–39, pp. 4, 35 (Hughes et al. 2006).

[29] Lucy Burke, 'Introduction: thinking about cognitive impairment', *Journal of Literary Disability*, 2.1 (2008), pp. i–iv (Burke 2008a); see also: Lucy Burke, 'Alzheimer's disease: personhood and first person testimony', presentation at the inaugural conference of the 'Cultural Disability Studies Research Network', Liverpool, May 2007, http://www.cdsrn.org.uk/Burke_CDSRN_2007.pdf (accessed August 2011); but no longer available (Burke 2007).

[30] Basting, 'Looking back from loss', p. 89 (Basting 2003); Cary Smith Henderson, *Partial View. An Alzheimer's Journal* (Dallas: Southern Methodist University Press, 1998) (Henderson 1998).

experience of dementia' that identified patient-authored narratives as a means to reclaim social and personal identity.[31]

The patient's as well as the caregiver's narrative will always give insight into the author-narrator's perceived difficulties with the condition; the losses experienced and the changes encountered. As such, they may be taken as confirming the stigma and fear existing in society. In setting my own work in the context of these original considerations, I argue that a shift in articulacy is strongly linked to political necessities and indicative of changes in societal notions of selfhood. Acknowledging patient narratives as such lifts the author-narrator onto a different level of authority; an act through which part of this identity-denying stigma is overcome and their advocacy is being heard. No narrative will embody such discernment relating to identity and the 'disruption of normal meaning-making activity' more acutely than the patient's *own* account.[32] If we were to keep overlooking the patient, the current cultural dementia narrative and its bearing on identity would remain solely informed by the caregiver-portrayed conception. In this context, the present work delineates correspondences and discrepancies between the caregiver's and the patient's perspective. This approach will illuminate the differences in the perception of identity in dementia. Recognition of the patient's continued identity, in turn, will impinge on healthcare and socio-economic decision-making as well as on the mainstream cultural image of the condition.

Conscientious Criticism: Mapping My Reading of Dementia Life-Writing

Illness narratives can never be representative of the population of individuals afflicted by a specific condition. This is particularly true in the case of dementia: while the number of patients voicing their experiences in writing barely rises above a dozen, most Alzheimer's disease narratives are authored by caregivers. Such caregiver deliberations, thus, primarily shape the general public's

---

[31] Ellen Bouchard Ryan, Karen A. Bannister and Ann P. Anas, 'The dementia narrative: writing to reclaim social identity', *Journal of Aging Studies*, 23 (2009), pp. 145–157, p. 147 (Ryan et al. 2009).

[32] I borrow this phraseology from John Wiltshire, 'Biography, pathography, and the recovery of meaning', *The Cambridge Quarterly*, 29 (2000), pp. 409–422, p. 413 (Wiltshire 2000) (see below p. 24).

perception of the illness. But in the awareness of the previously mentioned serious ethical implications pertaining to the understanding of identity and self in conditions of cognitive impairment, and in the light of the above-discussed implication of perceived dysnarrativia in Alzheimer's disease, we need to look beyond these caregiver accounts. We are urged to ask, whether they can reliably picture the patient's situation and world of experience, not least since the caregiver's agenda, inevitably, differs from the patient's outlook. We need to ask this question even in the awareness that patients themselves cannot write about their experiences in the final stages of the condition.

For example, Anne Hunsaker Hawkins's criticism focusing on the mythical conceptualisation of illness experience is highly relevant to a deeper understanding of dementia narrative. Amongst others, the patient's frequent allusion to their experience resembling a journey deserves close scrutiny for several reasons. According to Hawkins, 'the journey motif [...] restores to the ill person a sense of personal dignity and social value'.[33] At the same time, dementia is terminal and degenerative in nature and as such does, seemingly, not offer a possibility for the patient's 'insightful and enriched return'. And the caregiver's use of the journey myth, by comparison, matches, when for example thinking about Nancy Davis Reagan's deliberations on her husband's condition, the formulation of a completely different agenda.[34]

Set against these reflections, my study compares and contrasts third-person caregiver accounts and first-person patient autobiographies, particularly focusing – following G. Thomas Couser's example – on the poetical and political questions these narratives raise.[35] With respect to the

---

[33] Anne Hunsaker Hawkins, *Reconstructing Illness. Studies in Pathography, 2nd edition* (West Lafayette: Purdue University Press, 1999), p. 82 (Hawkins 1999).

[34] Martina Zimmermann, '"Journeys" in the life-writing of adult-child dementia caregivers', *Journal of Medical Humanities*, 34 (2013), pp. 385–397 (Zimmermann 2013b), and Zimmermann, 'Alzheimer's disease metaphors' (Zimmermann forthcoming).

[35] G. Thomas Couser asks similar questions; see: *Recovering Bodies. Illness, Disability, and Life Writing* (Madison: The University of Wisconsin Press, 1997), pp. 13–15 (Couser 1997); see also the reading strategies suggested in: Sidonie Smith and Julia Watson, *Reading Autobiography. A Guide for Interpreting Life Narratives* (Minneapolis: University of Minnesota Press, 2001), Chap. 7 (Smith and Watson 2001); of note, Couser recently published, again on caregiver narratives only: 'Memoir and (lack of) memory: filial narratives of paternal dementia', in *New Essays on Life Writing and the Body*, ed. by Christopher Stuart and Stephanie Todd (Newcastle upon Tyne: Cambridge Scholars Publishing, 2009), pp. 223–241, here and in the following

narrators' aesthetic choices it considers the following issues: what images do narrators appropriate and do they successfully formulate their myths; what narrative plot do they adapt; and how do they draw on established strategies of life-writing to support their telling. In the awareness that such poetic choices not only serve the narrators' private agenda but also their external presentation, I equally deliberate on how these accounts engage with the culturally dominant Alzheimer's narrative.

My reading of these texts will draw on narrative theory and work from anthropological and psychosocial sciences, and particularly address, how narrators negotiate with, and aspire to shape, the societal perception of the condition, and how their texts relate to discourses of gender, aging and disability. Ultimately, these reflections are permeated by deliberations on the distribution of power between patients and caregivers. More specifically, carers may well have the highly ethical intention to provide testimony and advice, but overlook – in devising coping strategies in the harsh confrontation with the relative's losses (about which the patient is no longer able to write) – the patient's remaining self and identity-affirming abilities. Such partial presentation, as we shall see, conditions the perception of patients as being passive and dissolving; characteristics that are not reconcilable with their own accounts of themselves.

These considerations directly relate to my concerns regarding the morality of 'regarding the pain of others', as Susan Sontag would say. Is there not a danger my background in neuroscience pushes my reading of dementia narratives towards being over-influenced by the cognitive limitations of their existentially and intellectually disabled narrators? And does my being removed from caring for an intellectually challenged individual put me in danger of reading these narratives not compassionately enough?[36] Such deliberations extend to the choice of texts discussed, not least as an added function of academic critique is – I am paraphrasing Arthur W. Frank here – to amplify voices and to connect them for enhanced strength.[37]

---

referenced from: http://www.academia.edu/8298268/Memoir_and_Lack_of_Memory_Filial_Narratives_of_Paternal_Dementia (accessed August 2016) (Couser 2009).

[36] On 'the split in critical attitudes' towards illness narratives, consider also: Ann Jurecic, *Illness as Narrative* (Pittsburgh: University of Pittsburgh Press, 2012), p. 3 (Jurecic 2012).

[37] In reviewing the highlights of the conference 'A Narrative Future for Health Care' (London, 19 to 21 June 2013), Arthur W. Frank's closing keynote emphasised the need for narrative medicine on both a practical and an academic level.

In view of the very limited number of patient narratives, I am considering accounts in English, French, German, Italian and Spanish literature, offering my own working translations in squared brackets in the running text. In this way, this study considers stories from the European, Australian and North American context. This approach may, at first sight, pose the difficulty that individual texts are not sufficiently considered within the specific cultural context from which they originate. However, it takes into account that both the incidence and prevalence of Alzheimer's disease and other dementias are particularly high in First World countries and that these nations all face similar socio-economic, healthcare and ethical challenges in the confrontation with the condition.[38] As such, I was not surprised to realise that there are clear, overarching narrative themes and recent developments that are consistently reflected in the presentation of both patient and condition across different languages and Western cultures.

In this respect, I am less concerned that this research could be biased as pertaining to what Sally Chivers deliberates upon, and Chris Bell calls 'White Disability Studies'.[39] Like its medico-scientific as well as humanities-related researchers, dementia, in general, and Alzheimer's disease, in particular, continue to belong, first and foremost, to the developed world – in terms of both their incidence and perceived burden.[40] These facts explain, in conjunction with Couser's deliberations on the non-representativeness of illness narratives, the phenomenon that dementia memoirs largely originate from the white middle-class background and, thus, necessarily dominate the array of narratives critiqued in the present study.[41]

---

[38] Sube Banerjee, 'The macroeconomics of dementia – will the world economy get Alzheimer's disease?', *Archives of Medical Research*, 43.8 (2012), pp. 705–709 (Banerjee 2012).

[39] Chris Bell, 'Is disability studies actually white disability studies?', in *The Disability Studies Reader, 3rd edition*, ed. by Lennard J. Davis (New York: Routledge, 2010), pp. 374–382 (Bell 2010); for further discussion, see: Sally Chivers, *The Silvering Screen. Old Age and Disability in Cinema* (Toronto: University of Toronto Press, 2011), p. 29 (Chivers 2011).

[40] On the perception of dementia in Eastern cultures, see, for example, John W. Traphagan, 'Being a good *rōjin*: senility, power, and self-actualization in Japan', in *Thinking about Dementia*, ed. by Leibing and Cohen, pp. 269–287 (Traphagan 2006), and Lawrence Cohen, *No Aging in India. Alzheimer's, the Bad Family, and Other Modern Things* (Berkeley: University of California Press, 1999) (Cohen 1999).

[41] Couser, *Recovering Bodies*, e.g., pp. 170, 183, 227 (Couser 1997); I have not come across published narratives by non-white caregivers or patients, but I point to recent work on the significant impact of race on caregiver experience in: Ilene C. Siegler et al., 'Caregiving,

Their small number as well as their insufficient analysis in a broader context has encouraged me to bring all patient accounts I became aware of during my studies into the present considerations: to the best of my knowledge, I have considered all popular press first-person accounts, including the print-on-demand texts available until 2013/2014 (though the number of print-on-demand texts steadily rises). By comparison, I had to choose which caregiver narratives to include in this consideration. Reading widely on the caregivers' plights and burdens, I realised that there are recurring themes in their telling, and these eventually suggested the structure of this book. Within these themes, I then selected texts that appeared particularly poignant or rich in their emphasis and presentation. Aiming to offer accounts of a diverse range of narrative forms and artistic expressions, I include memoirs, diaries, films, graphic novels, photo and picture books in my reading, and discuss them in relation to the limited existing scholarship on dementia narratives. I study textual narratives and visual material side by side, following Alan Radley's conviction that a focus on 'questions to do with serious illness, its understanding and the social response it provokes' allows for such comparative reading.[42]

Of course, the argument could now run that including patient blogs or interviews would significantly enlarge the sample. But I explicitly focus on accounts available on the book market, because, as for example Vai Ramanathan's dementia discourse analysis illustrates, depending on the audience we expect, we frame our story differently.[43] A blog may be freely accessible, but its primary audience is the intimate network of individuals confronted with similar experiences, so that much knowledge remains unsaid because it is already shared.[44] In writing for the general book market, author-narrators address a reader and publisher with a different set of expectations. This is partly related to the fact that – set against the transience of knowledge in the fast moving tweeting and chatting online world – a book allows for

---

residence, race, and depressive symptoms', *Aging & Mental Health*, 14.7 (2010), pp. 771–778 (Siegler et al. 2010).

[42] Alan Radley, *Works of Illness. Narrative, Picturing and the Social Response to Serious Disease* (Ashby-de-la-Zouch: Inkermen Press, 2009), p. 13 (Radley 2009).

[43] Ramanathan, *Alzheimer Discourse*, pp. 70, 125 (Ramanathan 1997).

[44] On electronic illness narratives as 'shared space', see: Arthur W. Frank, 'Illness and autobiographical work: dialogue as narrative destabilization', *Qualitative Sociology*, 23.1 (2000), pp. 135–156, p. 150 (Frank 2000).

the repeated return to its message, conveying stability, persistence and authority. In addition, as Arthur W. Frank puts it, published stories 'affect how others tell their stories, creating the social rhetoric of illness'.[45] At the same time, book publication demands an articulation sufficiently polished for communication aimed at political outreach. Tracing editorial efforts in a literary analysis brings home what it means to have to perform in what Stephen Post called a 'hypercognitive culture'; and additional meaning is uncovered where patients write against the cognitive norms that such a culture imposes. It is telling enough that several patient narratives have been self-published, that is, as print-on-demand, because they were not deemed polished enough by routine publishers.

The encounter in the hospital made me utterly aware of how abstract the condition is for all those who are not exposed to the daily encounter with the patient. Likewise, many policymakers are also removed from either experience – be it familial or professional caregiving. Convinced that illness narratives are the best teachers, where patient contact in the framework of hospital rounds or interviews is not easily achievable, I have included several of the narratives discussed here in my pharmaceutical care teaching.[46] Encouraged by the engaging response of students, I have become even more aware of the persuasiveness of these texts. Therefore, I hope that the present consideration of visual and textual narratives will offer their author-narrators an additional platform that reaches a readership beyond that which the original texts per se would and could achieve. Most of all, this book is meant to sharpen the politicians', health-economists' and care providers' eyes to the concerns of patients and caregivers. It seeks to contribute to the ongoing discussion regarding urgently needed changes in Western health-care systems that take into account the rapidly increasing numbers of individuals likely to develop symptoms of dementia.

For the purpose of these explorations, I specifically distinguish the notion of Alzheimer's disease, and dementia more broadly, from other brain damage insofar as the triad of incremental, chronic and untreatable

---

[45] Frank, *Storyteller*, p. 21 (Frank 1995).
[46] Martina Zimmermann, 'Integrating medical humanities into a pharmaceutical care seminar on dementia', *American Journal of Pharmaceutical Education*, 77.1 (2013), article 16 (Zimmermann 2013a); Ute Burkhardt et al., 'Literature and science: a different look inside neurodegeneration', *Advances in Physiology Education*, 36 (2012), pp. 68–71 (Burkhardt et al. 2012).

cognitive decline is the core threat in the Alzheimer's experience. In particular, I see a clear distinction between brain damage caused by events like a brain tumour, which usually involves very fast degeneration, a stroke, where the degenerative process is not experienced at all, or drug abuse, which implies self-inflicted brain cell death. By comparison, I am including – arguing from a neuroscientific perspective and understanding – narratives relating experiences with conditions very similar to dementia of the Alzheimer's type: Lewy body dementia that can co-present with Parkinson's disease, vascular dementia that may originate from transient ischemic attacks (TIA), and frontotemporal dementia. Put differently, I am looking at the type of degenerative chronicity that the cultural narrative links to the aging process, with Alzheimer's disease – unlike, for example, heart disease or arthritis – being much less medically accessible and physiologically tangible, but all the more threatening because it attacks the organ that is considered to harbour an individual's identity.

As a researcher on molecular mechanisms underlying acute and chronic neurodegeneration, I have been directly exposed to, and actively participated in the medico-scientific discourse regarding Alzheimer's disease for approximately fifteen years. As such, I am particularly aware that the current cultural dementia narrative is significantly structured by scientific and biomedical notions of the condition. These strongly relate to concepts of deterioration, decline, loss and death. But while I am conscious that I may be prone to reading dementia narratives through the medico-scientific lens, it will, at times, be necessary to appropriate the language of this neuroscientific narrative: I use medico-scientific terminology where narratives employ it, and also use this lexicon where I refer to medical and clinical aspects of the condition.

Mindful of Charles Riley's 'Guidelines for portraying people with disabilities in the media', my use of the term sufferer does not want to suggest that I perceive of each and every patient as suffering in and from their condition.[47] The life-affirming presentation of several patients clearly contests such biased reading. Still, a parsimonious use of this and similar expressions helps me to avoid persistent repetitions like 'individual with dementia'. Likewise, I define the caregiver as the spouse or adult child, who is closely exposed to the relative's condition, but not necessarily the

---

[47] Charles A. Riley II, *Disability & the Media. Prescriptions for Change* (Lebanon: University Press of New England, 2005), pp. 219–223 (Riley II 2005).

only or prime individual looking after the patient, even though both roles may coincide in the same person and author-narrator.

Sifting Dementia Narratives

The first part of this analysis, Chaps. 2 and 3, focuses on caregiver accounts. It asks how family members experience the condition – in relation to themselves as much as their parent or partner. I agree with Ann Burack-Weiss that memoirs do not lend themselves to an objective scrutiny of '[a]ge, gender, race, ethnicity, education, income, social class, religion, language, sexual orientation, and geographical location', since their author-narrators are self-selected.[48] Yet, core differences are present in terms of age and gender, not least, because caregiving, generally, continues to be considered the duty of the female, and the growing number of elderly patients imposes caregiving activities on adult children. Chapter 2 explores the direct impact on caregivers of being exposed to caregiving as such and, hence, the patient's decline on a daily basis. In this way, I hope to illustrate how the perceived degree of caregiver burden impacts on caregivers' understanding of themselves (as child or partner) as well as the presentation of the patient (as parent or partner). This analysis, by itself, will suggest the need for stronger socio-economic caregiver support.

At the same time, this chapter aims to separate out conceptual differences between parental and spousal caregiving and its impact on identity perception. This differentiation is necessary, because a 'history of reciprocity, along with a sexual history, separates the situation of partners from other family care relationships'.[49] I examine how shared memories of a life-long relationship colour patient presentation by the maintaining of pre-narrative identity. Parental caregivers, in turn, may well enter the caregiving experience in the aspiration to fulfil their generational duties, while – confronted with the loss of the parent – seeing their own identity as child at stake. I also argue that the increasing societal awareness of the condition and a related awareness of caregiver needs, also enabled

---

[48] Ann Burack-Weiss, *The Caregiver's Tale. Loss and Renewal in Memoirs of Family Life* (New York: Columbia University Press, 2006), p. 157 (Burack-Weiss 2006); consider, however, Diedrich's *Treatments* as a persuasive illustration of how illness narratives reflect wider cultural norms particularly related to class, gender and race (Diedrich 2007).

[49] Ibid., p. 69 (Burack-Weiss 2006).

by caregiver life-writing itself, led to a shift from a caregiver-centred to a more patient-centred approach in caregiving. This shift is strongly reflected in more recent caregiver accounts. If it is true that the reader's perception of the caregiver's moral stance is tied to the nature of patient presentation, this shift brings home the female caregiver's exposure to manifold ideological prejudices: expected hands-on daily care, personal experience of loss, struggle with personal identity issues and exposure to criticism for their so influenced narrative choices.

Chapter 3 further emphasises how the physical as well as emotional burden related to caregiving shapes patient perception. The usually less actively involved male family member has, thus, what I want to call a 'care-free' perspective on the patient and her/his condition. This chapter opposes the female perspective on caregiving to the male story. But it is less interested in identifying what it means to be the son or husband of a dementia patient as such. Rather, it seeks to detach the influence on the presentation of both illness and patient of the immediate caregiving experience and burden, specifically to illustrate the enormous psychological and emotional cost of treating a parent who is no longer a parent and how this particularly reflects on the presentation of the parent-turned-patient. In this way, it illuminates the impact on the perception of patient identity and the condition itself of cultural and socio-educational upbringing. More specifically, I argue that patient presentation is strongly gendered and closely related to societal attitudes to aging, and that enabling views of dementia emerge where aging is not considered merely in terms of loss. These insights reveal further working points for health-economists and policymakers.

In the second part of this analysis, Chaps. 4 and 5, I closely scrutinise patient narratives. Even though dementia first-person accounts are just beginning to take off in print-on-demand spaces, and the patient's voice has only been heard in a period scarcely exceeding twenty-five years, I sense phases of development reminiscent of the evolution G. Thomas Couser identified in the case of breast cancer narratives. Looking back on thirty years of life-writing, he identified that the 'genre' of breast cancer narratives developing in the 1970s had become removed from its initial impulses by the 1990s.[50] Similarly, and in agreement with Basting who identifies three phases in patient life-writing, I argue that the politicisation of dementia

---

[50] Couser, *Recovering Bodies*, p. 63 (Couser 1997); Diedrich made a similar observation, linking the rise of breast cancer narratives to the women's health movement of the 1970s and

narrative directly correlates with an increased societal awareness of the illness.[51] I will consider gender questions in relation to the author-narrator's advocacy for independence and autonomy, rather than scrutinising these narratives predominantly through the gender prism. In doing so, I will take stock of the small sociohistorical scholarship on Alzheimer's narratives that offers a reflective comparison between caregiver and patient life-writing set against social constructionist theories.[52]

Chapter 4 dissects how societal expectations regarding the patient's performance and productivity impose successful narrative articulation as central and integral to the perception of identity, social assertion and self. It explores how the first patient accounts develop coherent, linear narratives, and illustrates how the discrepancy between illness process and narrative plot impacts on the reader's perception of the condition. A comparative study of patient versus co-authored texts that additionally accounts for different stages in the severity of dementia will be as revealing as an analysis of sequential publications by the same patient. This investigation will support my argument that gradually intensifying patient activism enables patients' freedom of presentation, and, thus, begins to shift societal views on aging in general, and the condition in particular.

More recent Alzheimer's disease patient narratives take this activism further – in both form and contents: disease-imposed constraints become the narrative's core in terms of both aesthetic presentation and political pursuit. This development, mapped out in Chap. 5, thus, parallels the changes observed in caregiver life-writing, as patients and their needs reach the centre of narrative presentation and performance. I argue that patients can thrive, building on earlier advocacy of their fellow sufferers, on illness presentation that matches their attention span, live within their remaining abilities, and, thus, authoritatively claim their continued independence. This is especially the case for female patients who appear doubly strong when they overcome preconceptions of passivity and dependence – characteristics associated with cognitive impairment as much as being female.

---

politicisation related to the emergence of HIV/AIDS activism in the 1980s; see: *Treatments*, esp. Chap. 2 (Diedrich 2007).

[51] Anne Davis Basting, *Forget Memory. Creating Better Lives for People with Dementia* (Baltimore: The Johns Hopkins University Press, 2009), pp. 145–153 (Basting 2009).

[52] Jesse F. Ballenger, *Self, Senility, and Alzheimer's Disease in Modern America. A History* (Baltimore: The Johns Hopkins University Press, 2006), esp. Chap. 6 (Ballenger 2006).

My analysis, consequently, concludes with a consideration of the changes both caregiver and patient life-writing have gone through and how they mutually influenced each other. These changes have been conditioned by the rising number of individuals with dementia and the increasing societal presence of the disease. At the same time, these developments propelled forward a patient-centred movement, as more and more individuals touched by the condition aim actively to participate in shaping the mainstream dementia discourse. A deliberation on very recent third-person caregiver narratives will highlight how this evolution in patient perception has reached broader societal levels and promises to influence healthcare planning and socio-economic and cultural approaches to the condition.

In sympathetically analysing the testimony of those intimately affected by dementia, this book centrally contends that patient and illness perception and presentation develop within and impact on the evolution of dementia care and the appreciation of the patient's continued self away from the medico-scientific and health-economics dementia discourses. I believe the insights so gained to be accurate and dependable: dementia patient narratives are new enough to be free of 'second-hand' myths, as Hawkins calls them, and they are, as Couser would have it, more utilitarian than autobiographical in nature.

Open Access This chapter is distributed under the terms of the Creative Commons Attribution 4.0 International License (http://creativecommons.org/licenses/by/4.0/), which permits use, duplication, adaptation, distribution and reproduction in any medium or format, as long as you give appropriate credit to the original author(s) and the source, a link is provided to the Creative Commons license and any changes made are indicated.

The images or other third party material in this chapter are included in the work's Creative Commons license, unless indicated otherwise in the credit line; if such material is not included in the work's Creative Commons license and the respective action is not permitted by statutory regulation, users will need to obtain permission from the license holder to duplicate, adapt or reproduce the material.

CHAPTER 2

Of Wives and Daughters: Stereotypes of the Caring Female?

Abstract This chapter illustrates how the perceived degree of caregiver burden impacts on the caregiver's perception and, thus, presentation of the patient. The insights so gained call for stronger socio-economic caregiver support. 'Of Wives and Daughters' also aims to separate out conceptual differences between parental and spousal caregiving: shared memories of a life-long relationship colour patient presentation, also because they enable the maintaining of pre-narrative identity; daughters may care mindful of their generational duties, but see their own identity as child at stake. This chapter also argues that the increasing societal awareness of dementia and a related awareness of caregiver needs led to a shift from a stereotypical caregiver- to a more patient-centred approach in caregiving, which is strongly reflected in more recent caregiver accounts.

Keywords Adult child · Caregiver burden · Generational duty · Identity crisis · Parental loss

> First the mothers mother and then the mothers are mothered in turn.[1]
>
> Escribir este libro ha sido un intento más de acercarme a José Antonio desde su enfermedad [...]. Estas páginas son también un tributo a un amor desesperado [...]. Otro es el homenaje. Porque quiero que no se olvide la memoria de José [...]. También la solidaridad. Porque el dolor compartido es más útil y más llevadero [...]. Además, la rebeldía. Porque yo no estoy resignada [...]. Y la gratitud. Porque estoy en deuda con José Antonio.
>
> [Writing this book was a further way to stay near José Antonio since his illness (...). These pages are also a tribute to a love without hope (...). Another is homage. Because I do not want José's memory to be forgotten (...). Also solidarity. Because shared pain is more useful and bearable (...). Furthermore, protest. Because I am not resigned (...). And gratitude. Because I am indebted to José Antonio.][2]

In his review on pathographies, John Wiltshire illuminates our understanding of dementia as an illness that disrupts the pathographer's meaning of life. That he dedicates a third of his study to the analysis of the first two volumes of John Bayley's *Iris Trilogy* and Michael Ignatieff's *Scar Tissue* adds weight to his conviction that:

> diseases such as Alzheimer's [...] may well present the issues of identity which are implicit in all illness experience with particular acuteness. The need to create meaning, prevalent in the pathography in any case, becomes pressing when the patient, the very subject of the narrative, while apparently physically well enough, incarnates the disruption or bafflement of normal meaning-making activity, and seems in fact to be a different 'self' or to have lost the self that they were. The challenge of all illness experience may then perhaps be said to confront the pathographer of Alzheimer's with particular intensity.[3]

---

[1] Andrea Gillies in an interview following the publication of her memoir; see: Amelia Gentleman, 'The raw horror of Alzheimer's', *The Guardian*, 1 June 2010 (Gentleman 2010).

[2] Margarita Retuerto Buades, *Mi vida junto a un enfermo de Alzheimer* [My life next to an Alzheimer's patient] (Madrid: La Esfera de los Libros S. L., 2003), pp. 12–14 (Buades 2003).

[3] Wiltshire, 'Biography', p. 413 (Wiltshire 2000); Michael Ignatieff, *Scar Tissue* [1993] (London: Vintage, 1994) (Ignatieff 1994); unlike Wiltshire, scholars like Amelia DeFalco treat Ignatieff's text as fiction; see: 'Dementia, caregiving, and narrative in Michael Ignatieff's *Scar Tissue*', *Occasion: Interdisciplinary Studies in the Humanities*, 4 (2012), http://arcade.stanford.edu/occasion/dementia-caregiving-and-narrative-michael-ignatieff%E2%80%99s-scar-tissue (accessed August 2016) (DeFalco 2012).

Based on this fundamental insight, Wiltshire then explores the husband's (Bayley's) and the son's (Ignatieff's narrator's) difficulties to locate themselves in their relative's memory loss and unstructured behaviour. For example, with reference to Ignatieff's narrative, Wiltshire highlights formal aspects that reveal disturbance regarding boundaries of the self, pointing to 'the work's problematic status – evidently a memoir, but presented as a novel'. He also dismantles 'the present tense [as having] the effect of concealing [Bayley's] activity of recording, [which] is nevertheless the crucial goal towards which the narrator's energies are bent'.[4] Echoing Arthur W. Frank's description of the 'chaos narrative', Wiltshire's analysis asserts that the caregiver's ways of coping are mostly dependent on, even determined by, the patient, because the caregiver lives and acts in the awareness of the patient's imminent loss of self.

Wiltshire's argument seems to state the obvious, because it apparently resonates with what I have described as the cultural mainstream dementia narrative. But it has to be considered in the context of its time of publication. Offering a prompt reflection on Bayley's account, Wiltshire's was a much needed intervention on Alzheimer's disease in early dementia narratives.[5] Published at a time when caregiver issues only just began to enter wider societal awareness (amongst others, directly related to the publicity of Bayley's narrative), it perhaps unavoidably neglected potential differences in the spouse's as compared to the child's agenda. In addition, the study focused on illness experience more generally, rather than offering a detailed analysis of the 'recovery of meaning' in dementia caregiving.

This very recovery of meaning is my particular concern in the present chapter. I am interested in how caregivers deal with the condition and its consequences every day: what are their hands-on experiences, concrete challenges and unmet needs – from not being recognised by their own family member any more to the big question of when to place the patient into professional care. Knowledge so gained will inform policy discussions in its own right. But given that the sharing of their experiences by itself – their writing, drawing, photographing – is central to the caregivers' coping strategies, I particularly reflect on how they actually articulate their daily

---

[4] Ibid., pp. 419, 420 (Wiltshire 2000).

[5] I consider the first article by a literary scholar on 'Alzheimer's disease' narratives to be: Kathleen Woodward, 'Reminiscence and the life review: prospects and retrospects', in *What Does It Mean to Grow Old? Reflections from the Humanities*, ed. by Thomas R. Cole and Sally Gadow (Durham: Duke University Press, 1986), pp. 135–161 (Woodward 1986).

encounter with the patient: how do they interpret the illness's impact on their mutual relationship, and what images do they choose when writing about their family member. Such deliberations necessarily touch on issues as diverse as the ethics of patient presentation, the implications of the choice of narrative form(s) and the possibilities of varied artistic expression, with these issues requiring added reflection against the background of the increasing societal awareness of the condition over the last twenty years. Given then that caregiving continues to be seen as a predominantly female activity (despite a considerable shift within the 1990s that sees women's and men's involvement in caregiving converging), I initially, in this chapter, look at how daughters as compared to wives offer their stories.[6]

In particular, I illustrate that the adult child's choice of how she mythologises her parent's illness influences the child's own identity perception and, closely related, her presentation of the parent's personality. In my comparison of narratives by the writer Annie Ernaux and the women's studies scholar Carol Wolfe Konek, I argue that recreating the parent's pre-illness self has the positive effect of helping to preserve the own filial identity. However, this approach leaves no space for the parent's continued identity within the condition. Looking for personal growth in the confrontation with the parent's illness experience, by comparison, grants the parent the continued identity of a nurturing and teaching individual.

In the latter part of the chapter, I analyse how the history of a couple's life-long, shared relationship impacts on how a spouse faces her husband's illness. My reading of the narratives by Betty Baker Spohr, Judith Fox and Rachel Hadas also illustrates how creativity 'in an area of life where choice and creativity are almost wholly denied' structures the caregivers' understanding of their loss and the patient's increasing passivity through dementia.[7] Published across a time span of fifteen years, the aesthetic choices of a caricaturist, a photographer and a poet reflect a shifting conceptualisation of care away from caregiver- to

---

[6] Michael Hirst, 'Trends in informal care in Great Britain during the 1990s', *Health and Social Care in the Community*, 9.6 (2001), pp. 348–357, p. 354 (Hirst 2001); see also: Minna M. Pöysti et al., 'Gender differences in dementia spousal caregiving', *International Journal of Alzheimer's Disease*, article 162960 (2012) (Pöysti et al. 2012); they discuss: Kevin L. Baker and Noelle Robertson, 'Coping with caring for someone with dementia: reviewing the literature about men', *Aging & Mental Health*, 12.4 (2008), pp. 413–422 (Baker and Robertson 2008).

[7] Hawkins, *Reconstructing Illness*, p. 90 (Hawkins 1999).

patient-centred approaches. As observed in the context of filial accounts, these spousal tales also suggest that, where caregivers manage to perceive continuity, the patient's identity is preserved and the carer's burden appears less pronounced. Differently put, the female caregiver is exposed to manifold ideological prejudices. These include expected hands-on daily care, personal experience of loss, struggle with personal identity issues and also exposure to criticism for her so influenced narrative choices. My closing reflection on Reeve Lindbergh's narrative about her mother's dementia suggests that a patient can be considered active, and dementia may obtain added meaning, more easily in a 'care-free' environment whose wider cultural implications I then further explore in Chap. 3.

THE LOST IDENTITY: ALZHEIMER'S DISEASE, ADULT CHILDREN AND THE PAST

In a small volume of notes taken after visits to the nursing home, Annie Ernaux chronicles the final years of her mother's Alzheimer's disease.[8] Its most prominent feature is Ernaux's comparison of her mother to a child which becomes more and more explicit over time. Initially, she associates her mother's words with those 'I would use when I was a child' (15), later identifying her own gestures as those directed towards 'a child who is sleeping' (24), to approach the comparison of the mother to a 'frightened woman clinging to me like a child' (37). These periphrases, eventually, give way to the acceptance of their core truth: 'I help her to take off her panties and to put them back on. A child. Period' (53). Considering a diary as a place in which to contemplate one's self, Ernaux comes to 'learn some fundamental truth about myself' (29), namely, that, even though her mother now 'is my little girl [...] I CANNOT be her mother' (23; emphasis original).[9] Ernaux perceives the mother's condition and lost awareness of being mother as 'pushing me toward death' (63). In addition, she interprets

---

[8] Annie Ernaux, *Je ne suis pas sortie de ma nuit* (Paris: Éditions Gallimard, 1997); Engl. trans. as *I Remain in Darkness* (New York: Seven Stories Press, 1999) (Ernaux 1999); references from this English edition are incorporated in the text.

[9] Linda Anderson, *Autobiography* (Abingdon: Routledge, 2001), p. 35 (Anderson 2001).

the mother's cognitive changes as the accelerator of her aging and dying, which, in turn, threaten her identity as daughter.[10]

In this respect, the persistence and continuity of every diary entry defer the end of Ernaux's chronicling the mother's biography and her actual death, even though the literal plotting of her mother's decline necessarily brings her end ever nearer.[11] While this discrepancy strongly highlights Ernaux's emotional urgency, she nonetheless only published these fragments eleven years after her mother's death, as if to confirm our understanding of the privacy of such notes. In addition, the sequential presentation of differently accentuated accounts convincingly epitomises how continued caregiving may change the caregiver's attitude. French news presenter Françoise Laborde, for example, first relates personal feelings regarding her abrupt encounter with the mother's Alzheimer's disease, only later offering a more detached medico-clinical testimony.[12] Similarly, Mary Wilhoit kept a blog reporting the caring for her mother, which she only later published as a book. Asserting that a book makes her experiences more widely accessible, her writing as well as publication strategy nevertheless suggest she may be less sensitive to ethical issues: she reduces the patient to 'the mom [. . .] a mindless automaton roaming around' and posts to the blog while her mother is still alive.[13]

Ernaux's notes cannot, as Hawkins would have it, 'create a meaningful death', because her mother's style of dying did not reflect her actual personality.[14] This is perhaps a further reason why Ernaux initially composed, shortly after her mother's death, a narrative about her mother's life

---

[10] In an insightful analysis of Charles P. Pierce's narrative *Hard to Forget. An Alzheimer's Story* (New York: Random House, 2000) (Pierce 2000), Lucy Burke expands on how the adult child negotiates with the genetic risk of having inherited Alzheimer's disease; see: '"The country of my disease": genes and genealogy in Alzheimer's life-writing', *Journal of Literary Disability*, 2.1 (2008), pp. 63–74 (Burke 2008b).

[11] Susannah B. Mintz made similar observations for May Sarton's diaries; see: *Unruly Bodies. Life Writing by Women with Disabilities* (Chapel Hill: The University of North Carolina Press, 2007), Chap. 5, p. 186 (Mintz 2007).

[12] Françoise Laborde, *Pourquoi ma mère me rend folle* [Why my mother drives me crazy] (Paris: Flammarion, 2002) (Laborde 2002), and *Ma mère n'est pas un philodendron* [My mother is not a philodendron] (Paris: Flammarion, 2003) (Laborde 2003).

[13] Mary Wilhoit, *As She Was Dying. An Alzheimer's Journal* (Lincoln: iUniverse, 2008), p. 7 (Wilhoit 2008).

[14] Hawkins, *Reconstructing Illness*, esp. Chap. 4 (Hawkins 1999).

before dementia.[15] Its title, *A Woman's Story*, suggests detachment and distance, alerting the reader to the writer's search for form, in that 'the private diary is a practice [that] does not reflect the life as an autobiographical narrative would do'.[16] Ernaux follows the aspiration to be 'only the archivist' (15), and her use of bullet points reads as the author-narrator's acknowledgement of her limited knowledge of the mother's past. It is worth noting that the image of the archivist features in other adult-child life-writing, conveying feelings of loss in relation to the parent's own memory and life history, to which I return more fully in Chap. 3. Giovanna Venturino, for example, writes that:

> in modo inversamente proporzionale alla progressiva perdita di ricordi e conoscenze, la mia mamma estende sempre più il suo 'mare di nulla' dal quale, ogni tanto, come tristi relitti di un tempo ormai inesorabilmente andato, riaffiorano pezzi di ciò che è stata; e come uno scrupoloso, attento studioso, sono lì, pronta a raccoglierli [...].
>
> [In a way inversely proportional to the progressive loss of memories and knowledge, my mother increasingly expands her 'sea of nothingness', from which, every now and then, re-emerge, like sad relics of a time by now inescapably lost, pieces of all that she has been; and like a scrupulous and attentive scholar I am there, ready to collect them (...).][17]

The Italian primary school teacher's use of the archivist image suggests her perceiving of the mother's condition as one of a living death – both for its connection to the image of the 'sea of nothingness' and in its comparison to Ernaux's own use of the image. The French writer employs it to depict her activities after the mother's actual death. Specifically, Ernaux narrates, after having opened with the mother's death, the timeline of her life and dying. This construction closes the narrative circle, and mirrors – acknowledging the circle of life – the beginning of the daughter's healing.

---

[15] Annie Ernaux, *Une femme* (Paris: Éditions Gallimard, 1987); Engl. trans. as *A Woman's Story* (New York: Seven Stories Press, 1991) (Ernaux 1991); references from this English edition are incorporated in the text.

[16] Philippe Lejeune cited in: Smith and Watson, *Reading Autobiography*, p. 193 (Smith and Watson 2001).

[17] Giovanna Venturino, *Il tuo mare di nulla. La mia mamma e l'Alzheimer* [Your sea of nothingness. My mother and Alzheimer's] (Rome: A&B Editrice, 2012), p. 73 (Venturino 2012).

Ernaux, eventually, overcomes her clinging to the professed objectivity, 'to cry because she was my mother, the same woman I had known in my childhood' (80). These feelings, in turn, strongly resemble the emotional urgency that speaks from her original diary.

Ernaux is particularly aware of the intricate relationship between her act of writing – as a working through of her own past as daughter of a healthy mother and (much less) the years of the mother's illness – and her written words as a recreation of identity. In fact, the writer makes her narrative the counterstatement to what the disease did to her mother, as it 'puts my mother's illusory presence before her real absence' (88). It restores the mother to her original image, before dementia. At the same time, this act makes herself daughter again – a reading encouraged by insight that the female search for identity occurs 'through relation to the chosen other'.[18] In this awareness, it is most appropriate for Ernaux to publish the private notes, because they reflect a constituent part of her suffering.

The title of Carol Wolfe Konek's account *Daddyboy* similarly alerts the reader to the daughter's perception of the father's return to childhood.[19] But it also suggests how Konek, in distinction to Ernaux, continues to see the grown-up father through what she understands as childlike behaviour. This is particularly true, because the expression belongs to actual childhood conversations between 'Daddy's girl' and 'Daddyboy'. The use of this metaphoric oxymoron is particularly revealing compared to its usage in Nucci A. Rota's narrative of her mother's Alzheimer's disease. In affirming that, '[s]cendendo tutti i gradini della malattia è diventata quella che io ora chiamo la *bimbamamma*' [in descending all steps of the illness, she has become what I now call *mommy girl*], Rota professes the perception of her mother's 'other' personality through illness.[20] This reading underlines how Konek sees her father as a continued personality.

---

[18] Mary G. Mason, 'The other voice: autobiographies of women writers', in *Autobiography. Essays Theoretical and Critical*, ed. by James Olney (Princeton: Princeton University Press, 1980), pp. 207–235, p. 210 (Mason 1980).

[19] Carol Wolfe Konek, *Daddyboy. A Family's Struggle with Alzheimer's* (Saint Paul: Graywolf Press, 1991) (Konek 1991); references incorporated in the text.

[20] Nucci A. Rota, *La bimbamamma. Cosa vuol dire convivere con l'Alzheimer. Il diario di una figlia* [The mommy girl. What it means to share your life with Alzheimer's. A daughter's diary] (Naples: Iuppiter Edizioni, 2009), p. 17 (emphasis original) (Rota 2009); on the 'otherness' perceived in dementia, see: Ursula Naue and Thilo Kroll, '"The demented

Konek carries the title's antithetic message on a narrative level, when portraying the disruptive power of Alzheimer's disease by connecting different storylines, whose alternations do not follow a systematic pattern. The story of her growing up and being shaped by the confrontation with her father is interwoven with the story of her parent's progressing condition, as well as Konek's present-day dreams, her childhood thoughts and sections on the fear of losing her own self-awareness. Nevertheless, these storylines follow their individual timelines, suggesting that the narrator surrenders to her urgent need to maintain a sense of continuity that counterbalances her sense of biographical disruption.[21] This disruption is carried forward, as the patient's active presence decreases throughout the text, its second half reporting about him only from the distance of the third person, which mirrors involution and anticipates his death.

As Konek strings together snippets of past and present, her narrative resembles a series of photographs, each no longer than half a page told in the present tense. The father's 'gift to his family is history' (13), as he recorded memories through photography, a form which creates continuity, since Konek takes on the father's memory-making role. Just as the camera shoots one-moment-in-time images, she perceives of Alzheimer's disease itself as a condition that leaves room for no more than the current moment, when describing her father's attention, for example, as a 'flicker of knowing' (137). In this context, it is worth noting that Linda Grant's *Remind Me Who I Am, Again* similarly has the purpose of maintaining the mother's memory, as it describes her dementia which is caused by transient ischemic attacks, while recording the family's past, also in assembling photographs.[22]

In comparison to Ernaux, Konek continues to perceive of her ill parent as teacher, claiming that '[w]hen he had given all he could give consciously, he still gave us an example of endurance, of suffering, of awful mortality' (161). The very notion of continuity and closure reaches full circle, when, in her concluding lines, the daughter completely identifies herself with the father: 'I adored him. I worshiped him. I respected him. I judged him. I hated him.

---

other"': identity and difference in dementia', *Nursing Philosophy*, 10 (2009), pp. 26–33 (Naue and Kroll 2009).

[21] Michael Bury, 'Chronic illness as biographical disruption', *Sociology of Health and Illness*, 4 (1982), pp. 167–182 (Bury 1982).

[22] Linda Grant, *Remind Me Who I Am, Again* [1998] (London: Granta Books, 1999) (Grant 1999).

I accepted him. I pitied him. I released him. I become him' (161). This oscillating parallelism summarises the process *and* boon of Konek's working through the life-long father–daughter confrontation in the light of the father's illness. The negotiation with his condition becomes her opportunity for personal growth; an experience with lasting identity-shaping impact – as her choice to end the narrative with this statement in the present tense signals.

Read from this perspective, the informative wider societal purpose of Konek's work gains further meaning as she becomes the teacher herself. She lets us glimpse into support group meetings or scientific conferences, where the impression of medico-scientific and healthcare discourses that are insufficiently aware of caregiver burden prevails. As such, Konek's choice to report conversations with her mother – the primary caregiver of Konek's father – in direct speech furthers, in its perceived directness, the reader's appreciation of what society truly needs then and now: a discussion on the caregiver's pain and distress as well as the ethical considerations relating to end-of-life quality and care. Of course, the literalness of the words spoken must be questioned. But Konek would have been committed to maintaining fidelity to the gist of the conversations with her mother. As Sidonie Smith and Julia Watson point out, autobiographical narration 'cannot be read solely as either factual truth or simple facts. As an intersubjective mode, it lies outside a logical or juridical model of truth and falsehood'.[23] What is more, Barbara Ehrenreich appraises Konek's narrative as 'a powerful lesson about what it means to be human' on the book cover; the journalist's verdict being all the more meaningful in the light of her criticising the culture of survivor literature that leaves hardly any room for less triumphalist types of illness narrative.[24]

While Ernaux focuses predominantly on the daughter's self-survival in view of losing the parent to illness and death, Konek draws strong continuity within and beyond the parent's illness, likely in reverential love for the nurturing father.[25] Nonetheless, Konek is prepared to send the parent to a nursing home, with this decision often being supported by the societal

---

[23] Smith and Watson, *Reading Autobiography*, p. 13 (Smith and Watson 2001).

[24] Barbara Ehrenreich, *Smile or Die. How Positive Thinking Fooled America and the World* (London: Granta Books, 2010) (Ehrenreich 2010).

[25] On tensions in mother–daughter relationships, see: Ruth E. Ray, 'The uninvited guest: mother/daughter conflict in feminist gerontology', *Journal of Aging Studies*, 17 (2003), pp. 113–128 (Ray 2003).

concept of the career-oriented young mother. Andrea Gillies, for example, emphasises, as quoted above, generational duties, but eventually places her mother-in-law – conscientious of neglecting her own close family – in a care home. Konek's mother, in contrast, and spouses more generally consider caregiving as their obligation.[26] I, thus, turn to analysing three spousal accounts, whose different creative approaches per se suggest scope for improved, diversified caregiver support. They also highlight how a shared pre-illness experience (next to the parent–child relationship) structures the caregiver's perception of continuity or the loss thereof.

Times Are Changing: 'Mothers' and Lovers

Betty Baker Spohr's picture book traces her husband Hank's decline from diagnosis to death.[27] Every double page displays a pencil drawing and three to four paragraphs of related text that illustrates Spohr's confrontation with the illness in very short sentences, which hardly extend to a subordinate clause. Such a stylistic choice enhances the reader's impression that Spohr truly experiences her situation as an inescapable 'verdict' (1) – a metaphor that positions Spohr's illness experience close to the helplessness of Kafkaesque characters: it pictures her as being innocently, even arbitrarily, exposed to Alzheimer's disease, because '[t]he doctor's explanation leaves me in shock. There's no cure. There's no really effective medical help available. It's downhill all the way' (2).[28] The corresponding drawing shows the doctor in the dominant position: his big hand rests on Spohr's shoulder in the foreground of the drawing, while Hank himself – depicted with less attention to detail – is looking absentminded in the

---

[26] Neena L. Chappell and Valerie K. Kuehne, 'Congruence among husband and wife caregivers', *Journal of Aging Studies*, 12.3 (1998), pp. 239–254 (Chappell and Kuehne 1998); on the model of spousal caregiving as structuring later adult-child perception of duties, see: Liliana E. Pezzini, Robert A. Pollak and Barbara S. Schone, 'Long-term care of the disabled elderly: do children increase caregiving by spouses?', *Review of Economics of the Household*, 7.3 (2009), pp. 323–339 (Pezzini et al. 2009).
[27] Betty Baker Spohr with Jean Valens Bullard, *Catch a Falling Star. Living with Alzheimer's* (Seattle: Storm Peak Press, 1995) (Spohr 1995); references incorporated in the text.
[28] On Kafkaesque metaphors in relation to the patient's recovery after stroke, see: Martina Zimmermann, 'Narrating stroke: the life-writing and fiction of brain damage', *Medical Humanities*, 38 (2012), pp. 73–77, p. 74 (Zimmermann 2012).

background (3).²⁹ This text–picture portrayal suggests that Spohr perceives of the doctor as exercising his authority from a professional distance and with a mentality removed from the patient's as much as the caregiver's needs.³⁰

Spohr asserts that her writing and drawing 'turned out to be therapy for me' (iv) in the confrontation with feelings of:

> resentment that this dire thing should attack Hank [...]; self-pity as I began to have less and less freedom; guilt, fearing I was not doing enough [...]; embarrassment when he exhibited erratic, strange behavior; anger and impatience when he became impossibly stubborn [...]. (iii)

But her actual coping is rooted in her adopting 'an impersonal approach to my caregiving' (iv), which is reflected in her 'points to remember' that conclude each chapter. These points, for example, advise the reader to 'protect furniture and rugs, as if a baby were in the house' (200). As such, Spohr's detachment strategy goes hand in hand with her providing a narrative of largely informative nature that was, at the time of Hank's diagnosis around 1984, desperately needed: the only available manual was Nancy L. Mace's and Peter V. Rabins's *The 36-Hour Day*.³¹

Of course, in a first instance, the child metaphor saves her (as well as Ernaux) from writing about her husband's eating or toilet habits in the advanced stages of the illness. But while metaphors are part of explanatory models that 'enable sick persons to order, communicate, and thereby

---

[29] Allan Pease and Barbara Pease, *The Definitive Book of Body Language* (London: Orion, 2005), pp. 55–56 (Pease and Pease 2005).

[30] Rita Charon, *Narrative Medicine. Honoring the Stories of Illness* (New York: Oxford University Press, 2006) (Charon 2006); Kathryn Montgomery Hunter, *Doctors' Stories. The Narrative Structure of Medical Knowledge* (Princeton: Princeton University Press, 1991) (Hunter 1991).

[31] Nancy L. Mace and Peter V. Rabins, *The 36-Hour Day. A Family Guide to Caring for People Who Have Alzheimer Disease, Related Dementias, and Memory Loss*, 5th edition (Baltimore: The Johns Hopkins University Press, 2011) (Mace and Rabins 2011), first published in 1981 and then continuously re-edited; pictured by Spohr (210), who, thus, likely used this manual. Equally, Konek as well as the spousal caregiver Ann Davidson, in *Alzheimer's. A Love Story. One Year in My Husband's Journey* (Secaucus: Carol Publishing Group, 1997) (Davidson 1997), refer to it as the only manual, which further illustrates the need for shared reports. Spohr's conceptualisation of her ailing husband as being a 'different' personality, in turn, is likely influenced by the period's literature, namely, Donna Cohen and Carl Eisdorfer, *The Loss of Self: A Family Resource for the Care of Alzheimer's Disease and Related Disorders* [1986] (New York: W. W. Norton, 2002) (Cohen and Eisdorfer 2002).

symbolically control symptoms', they are also a mode of thought and, consequentially, action.³² In fact, Spohr identifies 'the man I married', to whom she dedicates her book, as 'slowly disappear[ing] as Alzheimer's disease inevitably took its toll' (iii). Following this detachment, she can draw even more disabling similes ethically, for example, picturing herself as putting a safe return bracelet around Hank's arm, while their little dog triumphantly lifts its paw (28), or showing Hank, next to their dog, confined by a baby-gate (104), as if to say that the patient needs more control and surveillance than the family pet. That Hank is usually depicted as slightly stooping further suggests Spohr's perception of his helpless inferiority.

Against this background, the most revealing statement remains Spohr's final confession that, suddenly, after Hank's death, her life is 'empty, without focus. For ten long years Hank has been the center of all my thoughts and activities. His illness has controlled every waking and sleeping hour' (208). Spohr's caring for Hank is her actual coping strategy that helps her not only to deflect the pain but also the awareness and anxiety about losing the husband himself; personal feelings for him cannot rise up, as he is being reduced to the mere origin of her caring strategies.³³

Reflecting on Spohr's need to provide testimony and offer advice to fellow caregivers makes one wonder how caregivers write about their experience – and, hence, portray their spouse – twenty years later. This question is pertinent, given how societal dementia awareness as well as caregiving approaches have changed since the 1990s. A recent caregiver manual, for example, summarises:

> studies have progressed from a focus [. . .] on the burdens of caring to research which focuses more on the interrelationship underpinning care giving and receiving [. . .], and more recently [. . .] where these interrelationships become the focal point for understanding the dynamics of living with dementia.³⁴

---

³² Arthur Kleinman, *The Illness Narratives. Suffering, Healing, and the Human Condition* (New York: Basic Books, 1988), p. 49 (Kleinman 1988); George Lakoff and Mark Johnson, *Metaphors We Live by* (Chicago: The University of Chicago Press, 2003), pp. 3–6 (Lakoff and Johnson 2003).

³³ Liora Navon and Nurit Weinblatt, '"The show must go on": behind the scenes of elderly spousal caregiving', *Journal of Aging Studies*, 10.4 (1996), pp. 329–342 (Navon and Weinblatt 1996).

³⁴ Charlotte L. Clarke et al., *Risk Assessment and Management for Living Well with Dementia* (London: Jessica Kingsley Publishers, 2011), p. 24 (Clarke et al. 2011).

Judith Fox's photo book illustrates such an altered caregiver attitude, as her work of art is, in witnessing her passion for photography and the continuing love for her husband Ed, much more autobiographical (rather than guide-like) in nature.[35] This insight is most clearly transported in a photo near the centre of the book (76). The couple's hands are portrayed, their wedding rings visible. As her fingers rest on his slightly blurred hand, which in itself signals Fox's metaphorical conception of Ed's decreasing presence, Fox pictures herself as the dominant part of the couple. But at the same time, this depiction tells the onlooker, '[i]n the midst of a devastating disease, [of] still lovely moments, laughs, hands held and bodies touched, and the precious and fragile gift of time together' (77).

Fox conveys a much more profound truth of the illness, because she documents, continuously changing her perspective, their life together against the background of Ed's gradual decline. A photo of Ed's naked back, cast into the striped shadow of the window blinds, conveys spells of insight and times of despair (49); a photo of Ed asleep taken from a distorting angle (suggestive of Andrea Mantegna's 'The Dead Christ'), hints at his increased vulnerability (90); a photo of Ed walking away from the photographer in the hallway of the house, implies his increasing disorientation (112); a photo of Ed taken from behind him and at a far distance in a hotel where the couple stayed, leaves the onlooker with the impression of the mere shadow of the patient (120). This series enhances the onlooker's understanding that the caregiver conceptualises the patient as 'fading away, becoming less and less capable of interacting with the world and with others in the ways he used to'.[36] In accord with these images that are so full of meaning – and in agreement with neurological insights regarding plateau phases in the illness trajectory – Fox writes:

> Once Ed and I started living with Alzheimer's, we began a trip down a never-ending staircase. Here and there we've found a platform and rested for a

---

[35] Judith Fox, *I Still Do. Loving and Living with Alzheimer's* (New York: Power House Books, 2009) (Fox 2009); references incorporated in the text; most of the photographs referred to in the following can be seen in a clip uploaded by Fox; see: '*I Still Do* by Judith Fox', https://www.youtube.com/watch?v=pWLhLD7Ox_g (accessed August 2016).

[36] Marya Schechtman, 'Getting our stories straight. Self-narrative and personal identity', in *Personal Identity and Fractured Selves*, ed. by Debra J. H. Mathews, Hilary Bok and Peter V. Rabins (Baltimore: The Johns Hopkins University Press, 2009), pp. 65–92, p. 71 (Schechtman 2009).

while. Then there was another step down. And another. Right now Ed and I are tumbling feet-over-head. No platforms in sight. A nightmare. (74)[37]

Like her photos, this journey language picks up on the general perception of Alzheimer's as leading to decline and darkness, and concomitantly expresses Fox's speechlessness in view of the disease process. But simultaneously, Fox pictures, in comparison to Spohr, the couple as being together in this descent, just as her work of art emphasises the close relationship between patient and caregiver, husband and wife, photo and text. The photos are able to tell the patient's story independently, while the text portrays – in addition to Fox's actual choice of perspective and sequence – the caregiver's awareness that:

> When we choose to help ease the life and death of an Alzheimer's sufferer, we are taking on a difficult, demanding, and heartbreaking role. And, yes, it's also a privilege. (80)

I believe this intricate combination of Fox being photographer, onlooker and carer as well as suffering partner all at the same time to be at the root of our perception that her work is devoid of any voyeurism; that, in fact, the beauty of these photos does not drain attention from their sobering subject.[38]

Undoubtedly, Fox's work does carry all this meaning, because it is deciphered against the background of twenty years of thoroughly informative caregiver writing; amongst others Konek's and Spohr's narratives. Indeed, her documentation gains additional connotations through the photos she does *not* show. She genuinely focuses on the coherent portraiture of the illness's impact on the couple's emotional as well as bodily relationship. This view is affirmed in Fox's concluding statement: 'Photographing the man I love is an intimate process' (124). Her work of art becomes a declaration of love to Ed, as is its title, since '[f]rom the moment we were married, he and I told each other daily, "I still do"' (125). Against this background, Fox's book essentially creates the continuation of the couple's life together beyond Ed's illness, because the photos will continue to speak to the onlooker Fox as they did to her as a photographer at the time. Fox records Ed in his living with the

---

[37] Edward Helmes et al., 'Patterns of deterioration in senile dementia of the Alzheimer type', *Archives of Neurology*, 52.3 (1995), pp. 306–310 (Helmes et al. 1995).
[38] Susan Sontag, *Regarding the Pain of Others* (London: Penguin, 2004), pp. 36–52, 68 (Sontag 2004).

illness, in his as well as her own suffering, affirming his personhood, continuing identity and self in Alzheimer's disease.

Confirming Elaine Scarry's discernment of the making power of art in the face of illness and pain, both Spohr and Fox find encouragement and strength in falling back on their passion for creative art work.[39] Rachel Hadas's recent memoir about her husband's dementia, in turn, offers precious insights into the support she gained from creative writing.[40] A closer scrutiny of the English scholar and poet's text also reveals that concepts of passivity – as they dominate Spohr's account, but are less prominent in Fox's book – do not categorically relate to a specific phase in dementia life-writing. They also emerge from a combination of the caregiver's aesthetic choices and the focus of her telling based on pre-illness experiences.

Having shared life-long intellectual companionship with the composer and professor of music, George Edwards, Hadas perceives of the condition as imposing increasing loneliness and isolation, writing that '[t]he pregnant silence of thinking [...] that hums with energy' (1) changes into '[t]he silence that came increasingly to reign in our house as George gradually changed from one person into another' (4). As such, her experience centres, as the narrative's title, *Strange Relation*, suggests, on the estrangement from, and the loss of, her partner in life, and, thus, the implications of being confronted with Alzheimer's disease in her own midlife.[41] Consequently, Hadas is less concerned with an illustration of George Edwards's pre-illness life or her hands-on caregiving experience. Rather, her telling expands on crossing her 'own private Rubicon' (75), that is, to call for household help, and, later, place her spouse into a nursing home. Her text makes this emotional turmoil

---

[39] Elaine Scarry, *The Body in Pain. The Making and Unmaking of the World* (New York: Oxford University Press, 1985) (Scarry 1985).

[40] Rachel Hadas, *Strange Relation. A Memoir of Marriage, Dementia, and Poetry* (Philadelphia: Paul Dry Books, 2011) (Hadas 2011); references incorporated in the text.

[41] Edwards and Hadas were sixty-one and fifty-six, respectively, at the time of diagnosis. Research is not clear on the difference in impact between early- and late-onset dementia, but particularly recognises high degrees of psychological suffering and specific problems related to the spouse's midlife; see, for example, Deliane van Vliet et al., 'Impact of early onset dementia on caregivers: a review', *International Journal of Geriatric Psychiatry*, 25.11 (2010), pp. 1091–1100 (van Vliet et al. 2010); Julie C. Lima et al., 'Spousal caregiving in late midlife versus older ages: implications of work and family obligations', *The Journals of Gerontology. Series B. Psychological Sciences and Social Sciences*, 63.4 (2008), pp. S229–S238 (Lima et al. 2008).

formally clear. George Edwards as an active partner in marriage appears absent; instead he becomes the reason for his wife's deliberations.

While her narrative stringently moves from diagnosis to institutionalised care, the entire central third of the text reminisces on the year 2007, the year before Hadas places Edwards into a care home. At its very centre, Hadas reflects on her poem 'The spell' (99), which 'focuses on one striking aspect of cognitive decline' (100), and, again, carves out the illness-imposed silence, as 'Your husband will remain /But scarcely ever utter one more word [...]. Within that garden henceforth, on each road, /Yours is the bearing of his lonely load' (100). Pondering her poem in *Strange Relation*, Hadas explains that she experiences the condition's cognitive aspects as most distressing, since, '[w]hen the person you're caring for is suffering from an ailment that affects cognition, there's twice as much to remember, to know, to keep track of' (101). Therefore, she concludes: 'The lonely load is he. Is his. Is mine' (102).

Like Ernaux, Hadas perceives of herself as 'the sole custodian of the fragile freight of George's past' (14), and her husband's 'archivist' (151) in the awareness of the illness-imposed 'open-endedness, this lack of closure' (168). Yet, this understanding helps her to approach the painful but necessary decision to place her husband into care. She retrospectively works through this choice reflecting on Richard Goodkin's description of 'the tragic middle':

> Tragedy tells us, as no other genre does, that even though not everything depends on us, even though we are acted on and constrained by forces beyond our control, nonetheless we must make unmakable choices. [...] The tragic middle recognizes not only that, as has been said of the tragic hero, you can't have it both ways, but also that you must have it both ways. (142)

Hadas's confession that through her personal experience of illness she 'came to understand tragedy as I never had before: from the inside' (24), acutely pinpoints how one's world of experience changes one's perception and, thus, representation of that very experience.[42]

---

[42] Hadas's strong emphasis on the title-suggested estrangement from her husband resonates with Janelle S. Taylor's deliberations on becoming 'stranger' in the relationship with her mother; the anthropologist's sharp insight that 'any medical institutionalization arguably entails a form of "social death"' further explains Hadas's perception of the tragedy in her situation; see: Janelle S.

In offering further readings of illness narratives within her own narrative of illness, in confessing that 'I found that poems were among my most faithful friends' (32), Hadas's text becomes yet another testament to how 'Readings in the Kingdom of Illness' (30) can become a haven of support and rescue. In this understanding, Hadas subsequently reminisces on her work in an article published in *The Lancet*:

> If silence was the enemy, literature was my best friend. No matter how lonely, frightened, confused, or angry I felt, some writer had captured the sensation [...]. I rediscovered what every writing teacher knows, that writing what you remember helps you to remember more. [...] the more I wrote, the more I remembered and understood. (ix–x)[43]

Her story testifies to the teaching powers of narratives and particularly emphasises, next to the personal, the political powers of narrative to participate in, and shape the mainstream dementia discourse.

Perceived Caregiver Burden and Patient Identity Condition Each Other

A core theme running through almost all of the above narratives is that the patient is compared to, or even presented as a child. Some adult children write, like Ernaux in her notes, under the spell of the daily parent-patient encounter. Others, like Konek, live at a long distance from their parent's home, seeing the patient only infrequently. Yet, their perception of the parent's childlikeness forms under the impression of a dementia discourse that continued, throughout the 1990s, to belong to the medico-scientific domain. This discourse particularly centred on caregiver burden, and identified similarities of the patient's to the child's brain organisation and behaviour.[44] It is assertions like these that Spohr's advice to 'expect regression to "second childhood"' (144) strongly resonates with.

Taylor, 'On recognition, caring, and dementia', *Medical Anthropology Quarterly*, 22.4 (2008), pp. 313–335, p. 320 (Taylor 2008); I am thankful to Jane Thrailkill for pointing me to this article.

[43] Rachel Hadas, 'Nothing's mortal enemy', *The Lancet*, 379 (2012), pp. 2142–2143, p. 2142 (Hadas 2012).

[44] Consider, for example, Alastair Burns, 'The burden of Alzheimer's disease', *International Journal of Neuropsychopharmacology*, 3 (2000), pp. S31–S38 (Burns 2000), and

We certainly could interpret Spohr's accepting the role of the accomplished coordinator as her continuing the husband's identity.[45] This perspective would put her coping strategy on one level with those pursued by adult-child caregivers who seek continuity in their living up to the role of the parenting child and, in this way, substitute the parent. Such strategies may prove useful in the short term, but leave the caregiver confronted with identity struggles after their family member's death, as both Spohr's narrative and Ernaux's notes testify. In addition, such patient conceptualisation may quickly structure how patients and their care are confronted. An annotated bibliography on *Literature and Gerontology* published in the mid-1990s illustrates my concern. While such work offers an overview on less well-known narratives related to mental health and dementia in old age, the list of relevant narratives is – with a view to the bibliography's publication date – rather short, and omits a clear distinction between fictional and non-fictional texts. Yet, the authors emphasise patients as being 'shown as repulsive to those attending to them [...who] often feel embarrassed by their bizarre, unpredictable behaviors'.[46]

Fox, in comparison, writes against the background of a changing conceptualisation of dementia care a decade later, and was, given that she acknowledges Lisa Snyder's work, certainly influenced by literature on the biopsychosocial approach to dementia and caregiving.[47] In exploring the nature of personal identity through the prism of philosophy and psychiatry, such research identifies, as highlighted in the introduction, patients as able to maintain their feelings of self-worth. That Hadas's patient image, by comparison, lingers on concepts of loss, silence and absence at a time when these whole-person approaches had already made headway underlines how

---

Carl-Otto Jonsson et al., 'Exploratory behavior in patients suffering from senile dementia: a comparison with children', *Acta Psychiatrica Scandinavica*, 53.4 (1976), pp. 302–320 (Jonsson et al. 1976). For an overview of scientific insights that have been collected regarding these issues, see: David Shenk, *The Forgetting. Alzheimer's: Portrait of an Epidemic* (New York: Anchor Books, 2003), pp. 121–130 (Shenk 2003).

[45] Toni Calasanti and Mary E. Bowen, 'Spousal caregiving and crossing gender boundaries: maintaining gendered identities', *Journal of Aging Studies*, 20 (2006), pp. 253–263 (Calasanti and Bowen 2006).

[46] Robert E. Yahnke and Richard M. Eastman, *Literature and Gerontology. A Research Guide* (Westport: Greenwood Press, 1995), p. 35 (Yahnke and Eastman 1995).

[47] Lisa Snyder, *Speaking Our Minds. What It's Like to Have Alzheimer's* [1999] (Baltimore: Health Professions Press, 2009) (Snyder 2009).

shared pre-illness experience structures illness and patient perception. Ernaux's experience is structured by the loss of the nurturing mother, Hadas's by the loss of intellectual companionship. Consequently, their presentations appear dominated by concepts of the patient's passivity.

In this context, an analysis of allusion to performance within the narratives discussed above proves insightful especially with a view to their choice of humorous presentation. In my undergraduate teaching, the two drawings by Spohr referred to above elicited most animated discussion, particularly, with respect to the ethicality of such presentation. Many students perceived of their humour as funny at the expense of the patient – even though it might help Spohr's survival, since deflecting stress from the daily strain of caregiving. Still, such presentation is in stark contrast to Fox's portrayal of Ed as keeping (as the patient himself) his humour and wit even in the face of disease progression. Offering a photograph of Ed looking into the mirror, pulling a face and sticking his tongue out (53), Fox asserts:

> Laughter allows Ed to feel normal and it deflects attention away from the fact that he might not be able to answer the question, recall the name, or find his way to the front door. (52)

Pushing an analysis of performance in dementia life-writing further suggests, how strongly the freedom from caregiving – or, more generally speaking, the caregiver's perceived situation (thinking about the lover Fox as compared to the 'mother' Spohr and the abandoned companions Hadas and Margarita Retuerto Buades, whom I cite above) – both builds on and prepares for the perception of the patient's condition, behaviour and identity. In fact, we might perceive of Fox's patient conceptualisation as more active because of Ed's lived presence in the photographs, and because we look at these pictures in the context of Hadas's choice to let her account be structured by George's increasing cognitive absence. I want to illustrate this important relationship further by briefly looking at Reeve Lindbergh's memoir of her mother.[48] One is immediately touched by Lindbergh's lyrical account and could read it as a poetic rendering of her mother's

---

[48] Reeve Lindbergh, *No More Words. A Journal of My Mother, Anne Morrow Lindbergh* [2001] (New York: Touchstone, 2002) (Lindbergh 2002); references incorporated in the text.

dementia. Yet, I particularly want to focus on Lindbergh's attention to her mother's behaviour and related choice of presentation.

After a series of strokes several years earlier, Lindbergh's mother is left mentally confused and, as the narrative's title, *No More Words*, anticipates, unable to speak.[49] Reeve Lindbergh suffers 'in silence', not 'know[ing] what to do with her [mother]. It is the silence. [...] I am bewildered, confused, absolutely at sea, in my mother's silence' (14). She shares this experience with her friend Hadas, and particularly empathises with Hadas being confronted with George Edwards's 'living absence and an almost total silence'.[50] In her own narrative, Lindbergh describes her suffering in the confrontation with silence as follows:

> To lose such an important listener in life is like losing my shadow. With no shadow, does a person truly exist under the sun? With no listener, does a person really have a voice? Silence means so many things to human beings. Some of them are unbearable. (85)

To fill this void – and certainly also in the need to keep the parent's memory – Lindbergh quotes the mother's work throughout her memoir. At the same time, she comes to the conclusion that:

> Language is limited at the best of times. What really goes on in this world is beyond words, and the truth of it, whatever that is, comes through to us in mystery, always taking its own sweet time. (135)

In this conviction, Lindbergh places noticeable emphasis on the mother's remaining actions, reminiscent of Konek's attempts at seeing the still teaching father. Additionally, she stresses her own desire to interpret the mother's behaviour in particularly active terms, even though the couple spends most evenings sitting together in silence. On one such evening, the former pilot takes her daughter by surprise, while holding on to a cuddly toy:

---

[49] Even though the pilot's condition appears to originate from a stroke, I choose to consider Reeve Lindbergh's narrative here, because Anne Morrow Lindbergh's dementia is presented as age-related cognitive decline, with the publisher advertising the narrative's relevance to those 'who care for an elderly parent disabled by Alzheimer's or stroke' on the book's back cover.

[50] Lindbergh's praise for Hadas's narrative; see: Hadas, *Strange Relation*, p. i (Hadas 2011).

> Holding it, she watched me for a while, then put down the mouse and picked up a glass of water. She turned the glass over and poured it on my knee. *I don't care what they say about short-term memory loss. She's been planning that for a week.* (108; emphasis original)

In reference to an earlier scene, where her mother poured grapefruit juice from a glass into a vase with lilies, Lindbergh tells us that she tries to interpret her mother's behaviour as purposeful action, identifying streams of thought. Thus, Lindbergh concludes: 'Liquids are for pouring. So she poured' (109). In the same way, the daughter reflects humorously on how her mother apparently objects to her toes being treated by the podiatrist, who eventually gives her a catalogue, with which the mother bops him on the head, but only:

> when he was working on a particularly hard or tenacious nail. The gesture was almost regal. *I dub thee Sir Arthur, Knight of the Protested Pedicure.* He clipped, she bopped, I watched. (134; emphasis original)

This final parallelism – reduced to subject and predicate just like the short factual statement above – suggests Lindbergh's role as that of an onlooker in her mother's continued activity, which, however, is reduced to minimal actions. Both scenes leave us, especially in the light of Lindbergh's jokey commentary, with the impression of the mother's happily tolerated, even appreciated, childlike mischievousness. In fact, Lindbergh's allusions to buying an 'anthology of poems and prayers for children' (82) or a book 'in the format of a coloring book for children' (127) for her mother let us appreciate a much more relaxed use of the child metaphor than that seen in Ernaux's or Spohr's account.

Humour in adult-child caregivers has been identified as being closely related to the caregiver's general perspective on life as well as the parent's own nature.[51] This explanation certainly fits Reeve Lindbergh's situation, when considering the strong Buddhist imprint in the mother's actual caregiver environment. Yet, I believe that Lindbergh is particularly able to picture her mother's condition with a pinch of laid-back rather than

---

[51] Tracy Tan and Margaret A. Schneider, 'Humor as a coping strategy for adult-child caregivers of individuals with Alzheimer's disease', *Geriatric Nursing*, 30 (2009), pp. 397–408 (Tan and Schneider 2009).

black humour (as Spohr's seems to remain), since she is writing from a 'care-free' distance:

> Mother does not live in my house, but in a smaller one [...], only a hundred yards away. I visit her in the evenings, but full-time caregivers keep her company twenty-four hours a day. They help her eat and dress, and tend to her bathing and personal care. (14)

But even when taking into account this caregiving relief, I am aware that I here offer a rather sympathetic reading of Lindbergh's attempts to keep her mother alive and active, and am wondering why I see Lindbergh's alluding to perceiving of her mother as a child with such serenity. Am I interpreting her rendering in much more positive terms, because I have her open acknowledgement 'that Mother is very fortunate to be able to afford such care, and that I am very fortunate to have her near – but not in – my home' (14)? Given that the issue of gender is part of how we read a narrative, I wonder whether we absorb Fox's photo book, Lindbergh's memoir or even Spohr's account – which is, after all, written in the emotional turmoil of losing the beloved husband – with deeper involvement as they are told by a woman, with whom I, as a gendered reader, might in addition identify more fluidly.

I first became invested in this question, when studying fictional accounts centred on dementia caregiving, and felt particularly drawn into deliberations on such predetermined reading where author and narrator, alias main protagonist, had the same sex.[52] I believe this question to be particularly pressing, given that the female perception of their ailing relative – and, thus, their choice of illness and patient presentation – may significantly differ from male approaches, not least since men are rarely primary caregivers and, additionally, rather define themselves autonomously. In addition, the number of female narratives significantly exceeds that of male accounts, which may be rooted in the fact that men find it difficult to maintain their sense of masculinity in the feminine role of caregiving or

---

[52] Martina Zimmermann, 'Deliver us from evil: carer burden in Alzheimer's disease', *Medical Humanities*, 36 (2010), pp. 101–107 (Zimmermann 2010), and therein: Susan S. Lanser, 'Queering narratology', in *Ambiguous Discourse: Feminist Narratology and British Women Writers*, ed. by Kathy Mezei (Chapel Hill: The University of North Carolina Press, 1996), pp. 250–261 (Lanser 1996).

indeed after having published an account of caregiving.⁵³ These caveats suggest that the female author-narrator may be exposed to a range of ideological preconceptions that are enhanced by the caregiving experience and its representation. Mindful of these circumstances, I want to turn, in the next chapter, to several narratives written by male caregivers.

Having identified scope for healthcare and economic changes in this first chapter – an alleviation of caregiver burden will impact on patient identity perception, even though a life-long shared experience will enhance feelings of loss and passivity – I am now turning to sociocultural implications of altered caregiver circumstances. In juxtaposing the male to the female narrative in the following chapter, I am looking for notions of the patient and condition that might only come to the fore, once the caregiver-narrator is able to write from a distanced breathing space, removed from the imminent day-to-day impression and burden of caregiving – as possibly suggested in Lindbergh's 'care-free' descriptions. This means, I am less interested in the difference between the male and female experience of looking after a family member with dementia as such. Rather, this approach will illustrate in more detail the enormous emotional strain on children who have to care for a parent who is no longer their parent. It will also show that the specific meaning of memory is embedded in a particular personal background and upbringing as well as a wider cultural and historical tradition. Building on insights gained so far, such meanings will only change – losing connotations of stigma and fear – with a shift in caregiver burden.

---

[53] Oscar Ribeiro, Constança Paúl and Conceição Nogueira, 'Real men, real husbands: caregiving and masculinities in later life', *Journal of Aging Studies*, 21 (2007), pp. 302–313 (Ribeiro et al. 2007); Jeanne Hayes, Craig Boylstein and Mary K. Zimmerman, 'Living and loving with dementia: negotiating spousal and caregiver identity through narrative', *Journal of Aging Studies*, 23 (2009), pp. 48–59 (Hayes et al. 2009); Ad J. J. M. Vingerhoets and Guus L. van Heck, 'Gender, coping and psychosomatic symptoms', *Psychological Medicine*, 20.1 (1990), pp. 125–135 (Vingerhoets and van Heck 1990); see also Couser's observation on the demographics of the writers and written-about, in 'Memoir and (lack of) memory', pp. 3–4 (Couser 2009).

Open Access This chapter is distributed under the terms of the Creative Commons Attribution 4.0 International License (http://creativecommons.org/licenses/by/4.0/), which permits use, duplication, adaptation, distribution and reproduction in any medium or format, as long as you give appropriate credit to the original author(s) and the source, a link is provided to the Creative Commons license and any changes made are indicated.

The images or other third party material in this chapter are included in the work's Creative Commons license, unless indicated otherwise in the credit line; if such material is not included in the work's Creative Commons license and the respective action is not permitted by statutory regulation, users will need to obtain permission from the license holder to duplicate, adapt or reproduce the material.

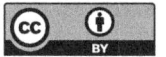

CHAPTER 3

From a 'Care-Free' Distance: Sons Talking About Cultural Concepts

Abstract The usually less actively involved male family member has what I call a 'care-free' perspective. In analysing narratives by sons, this chapter seeks to detach the influence on illness and patient presentation of the immediate caregiving experience and burden. Less interested in identifying what it means to be the son or husband of a patient as such, this chapter specifically illustrates the enormous psychological and emotional cost of caring for a parent who is no longer a parent. In this way, it illuminates the impact of cultural and socio-educational upbringing (rather than daily caregiving) on the perception of patient identity and the condition itself. It argues that identity-affirming patient presentation is strongly gendered and closely related to societal attitudes to aging.

Keywords Aging · Continued personhood · Educational background · Intellectual abilities · Pre-illness identity

> Now that she can no longer be hurt by me, by her family, by those who knew her, by any of us, surely I may open her letters and use them to help tell her story? But I hear my father's warning: 'Please remember that one day someone may have to write your biography'.[1]
>
> I began to think of my mother as a philosophical problem.[2]

As one of the first pieces of literary criticism regarding dementia narrative, Kathleen Woodward in 1986 focused our attention on the impact of dementia as a debilitating condition in old age.[3] Her comparative analysis concentrated on a son's memoir, Yasushi Inoue's *Chronicle of My Mother*, and a journalist daughter's feature story published in the *New York Times Magazine*.[4] In placing her analysis in the context of deliberations on the representation of old age, her work draws important attention to the fact that present-day society perceives changes in cognitive processes intricately to be linked to, even synonymous with, older age. Dementia has begun to epitomise the sum of illness, aging and dying.[5]

One of the core merits of Woodward's insights is that it alerts the reader to the fact that the representation of dementia must be dissected in connection with a consideration of the societal repulsion of aging. In this respect, Susannah B. Mintz's recent analysis of May Sarton's journals strongly echoes Woodward's views, when it reveals how 'physical and cognitive shifts associated with aging become the unacknowledged, because feared, potential of human corporeal existence'.[6] Additionally, in comparing a text authored by an American journalist to that of a Japanese author, Woodward's work develops a clear understanding of how the specific meaning of memory and its loss are produced within particular historical settings and cultural beliefs. Given the scarcity of narratives available at the time of publication however, Woodward could not explore how different cultural settings,

---

[1] Michael Holroyd, *Basil Street Blues. A Family Story* [1999] and *Mosaic* [2004] (London: Vintage, 2010), p. 144 (Holroyd 2010).

[2] Ignatieff, *Scar Tissue*, p. 53 (Ignatieff 1994).

[3] Woodward, 'Reminiscence and the life review' (Woodward 1986).

[4] Yasushi Inoue, *Chronicle of My Mother* [1975; trans. 1982] (New York: Kodansha America, 1985) (Inoue 1985); Marion Roach, 'Another name for madness', *New York Times Magazine*, 16 January 1983 (Roach 1983).

[5] O'Rourke, 'Alzheimer's disease as a metaphor' (O'Rourke 1996).

[6] Mintz, *Unruly Bodies*, p. 183 (Mintz 2007).

educational backgrounds and the upbringing in a specific environment shape how caregivers confront dementia in their family member. In its scope, Woodward's work also neglects the influence on patient presentation of the parent's life history and life-long role in the adult child's nurturing – aspects that involve a discussion of gender and aging in relation to patient presentation. These are my concern in the present chapter.

In looking at narratives by male rather than female caregivers, I hope to factor out the impact on representation of the burden of daily care. Apart from John Bayley's narrative, I came across only one other account written by a male spouse. Like Betty Baker Spohr, Frank Wall provides a candid guide-like account, based on the idea that 'two Marys were created', which further supports my hypothesis that caregiver burden per se overwrites gender-related patient conceptualisation.[7] Of course, following Shirley Neuman, we might read Wall's detachment as professionally male, while perceiving of Spohr's as a deliberate injunction against 'the personal, intimate' of female autobiography.[8] That said, given the compelling similarities regarding disease and patient presentation in, and the time of publication of, Wall's and Spohr's texts, I here reflect rather on several adult-son accounts. Their discussion, however, demands a consideration of the best known and most frequently cited of all Alzheimer's narratives: John Bayley's narratives about his wife, the British writer and philosopher Iris Murdoch. Especially *Iris: A Memoir of Iris Murdoch* continues to provide inspiration, and at times moral justification, for other caregivers, among them (as referred to in Chap. 2) Margarita Retuerto Buades, Andrea Gillies and Nucci A. Rota, as well as David Sieveking, whose film I analyse in the conclusion to this book.

My analysis will, first and foremost, look at the author-narrator's illness and patient presentation as shaped by the life-long relationship between parent and child; this relationship influences the choice of metaphors; the importance assigned to losses as compared to gains; and the meaning ascribed to the parent's illness as such. As previously, knowledge so gained will directly inform policy discussions, because the familial caregiver is able to see lifetime continuity and can encourage identity-affirming care that respects the patient's past experiences and achievements.

---

[7] Frank Wall, *Where Did Mary Go? A Loving Husband's Struggle with Alzheimer's* (Amherst: Prometheus Books, 1996), p. 142 (Wall 1996).

[8] Shirley Neuman, 'Autobiography and questions of gender: an introduction', *Prose Studies*, 14.2 (1991), pp. 1–11, p. 2 (Neuman 1991).

In the first part of this chapter, I illustrate how children's perception of the parent's role in their upbringing influences their writing about them once they have dementia. My comparison of narratives by the German journalist Tilman Jens and the Canadian photographer Jean Grothé argues that writing about a parent whose intellectual prowess dominated the son's life unavoidably centres on the parent's cognitive losses. Illustrating the illness of a life-long nurturer, by comparison, may be more focused on the parent's aging as such. This discussion necessarily reflects on the role of the parent's gender, because, in our cultural hermeneutics, females have been associated with the nurturing body and concepts of dependence and vulnerability: they are 'linked with nature, sexuality, and the passions, whereas men have been identified with the rational mind'.[9] Reading these narratives against John Bayley's account reveals that awareness of the patient's life history and achievements overwrites a gendered rendering of the illness.

Having established the crucial role of parents' life history for their representation, I turn to the link between Alzheimer's and aging more fully in the second part of this chapter. I argue that positive notions of aging, including concepts of wisdom and life-experience, can structure those of dementia and influence identity affirmation. The photographs of the Italo-American Phillip Toledano and the writings of the Austrian Arno Geiger reflect the enabling powers of patient appreciation. In contradistinction to Chap. 2, my analysis explicitly focuses on the perception and presentation of the patient, not the identity crisis of the child. But it will become clear that patient affirmation feeds back into the adult child's own wellbeing: it influences perception of continued identity as a child. My closing reflection on Josh Appignanesi's autobiographically inspired short film *Ex Memoria* channels considerations on the patient's life history and old age towards a deliberation on the patient's own perspective particularly in an identity-denying healthcare environment. This discussion prepares the ground for a closer scrutiny of patients' own writings in Chaps. 4 and 5.

---

[9] Drew Leder, *The Absent Body* (Chicago: The University of Chicago Press, 1990), p. 154 (Leder 1990); see also: Michelle Fine and Adrienne Asch, 'Introduction: beyond pedestals', in *Women with Disabilities: Essays in Psychology, Culture, and Politics*, ed. by Michelle Fine and Adrienne Asch (Philadelphia: Temple University Press, 1988), pp. 1–37, pp. 3–4 (Fine and Asch 1988).

Body and Mind: The Patient as Object

Both on a textual and a narrative level, John Bayley looks for shared continuity in the couple's life together under the spell of Alzheimer's disease.[10] Incessantly, he reformulates motifs that were important in the couple's past – like swimming in the river, and water in general. Their contextualisation in the present emphasises the life-changing impact of the condition, when Bayley, for example, states that their 'communication seems like underwater' (41). To describe the lingering in memories of his own childhood, he depicts himself as '[s]ailing my little boat slowly down the stream of memories' (271). This expression, in turn, picks up on Murdoch's own assertion of 'sailing into the darkness' (194). It also hints at the husband's attempt to make their experiences mutual: their frequent loss of understanding, their silence in front of the other.

In line with this observation, the most striking symbol for attempted continuity reveals itself in the way Bayley praises 'the joys of solitude' in their marriage, meaning '[t]o be closely and physically entwined, and yet feel solitude's friendly presence' (94). Only a few pages later, the scholar admits:

> Now we are together for the first time. We have actually become, as is often said of a happy married couple, inseparable [...]. It is a way of life that is unfamiliar. The closeness of apartness has necessarily become the closeness of closeness. And we know nothing of it; we have never had any practice. (96)

These different notions of silence and solitude resonate with Hadas's experience of lost companionship. But in comparison to the American poet, the British writer zeroes in on the raw fact that Iris is not able to choose her lifestyle; that her former independent lifestyle has turned into full dependence on Bayley and his care.

Bayley transports the momentous nature of this disease-imposed transformation on a textual and narrative level: the second, much shorter part of his account is composed of diary-like entries in the present tense. They tell about the challenges of daily care, and employ images that convey

---

[10] An earlier version of this chapter has been presented at a workshop on 'Medical Humanities and Aging', King's College London, 10 December 2014.

Murdoch's dependence on Bayley. Amongst others, we read about the couple's 'child talk', and gather that:

> She never showed any interest in children before. Now she loves them, on television or in real life. It seems almost too appropriate. I tell her she is nearly four years old now – isn't that wonderful? (201)

As previously mentioned, Bayley's narrative has obtained its prominence in conjunction with Richard Eyre's movie adaptation: both critical reception and didactic use of his memoir have been aided by the film's outreach and message.[11] Yet, the film is considered 'to transform Iris Murdoch into a mascot for dementia'.[12] This fact might have supported professional interest in the movie.[13] But it also favoured the almost undisputed use of Bayley's narrative to illustrate how the illness reduces the patient not only to a child but also to a living death. With reference to Paul John Eakin's assertion that Alzheimer's represents 'the death of the self', Lisa Diedrich, for example, writes that '[i]n the case of Bayley's narrative of Murdoch, the first death is the death of the self through Alzheimer's that precedes the death of the biological body'. Diedrich puts her claim specifically in the context of Murdoch's achievements as a philosopher and novelist. As such, one could argue that in Murdoch's case the loss of self becomes particularly apparent, because the reader reflects on her illness in the light of her past achievements, or, as Diedrich puts it: 'Bayley's task [...] is to describe what happens [...], but, in describing the losing that occurs with Alzheimer's, he must also describe that which has been lost'.[14]

---

[11] For example, Bayley's trilogy and Eyre's film set the end point in the 'Illness narrative as life writing' seminar series at King's College London in 2010/2011; they also featured in my own graduate seminar series; see: Burkhardt et al., 'Literature and science' (Burkhardt et al. 2012).

[12] Amelia DeFalco, *Uncanny Subjects. Aging in Contemporary Narrative* (Columbus: The Ohio State University Press, 2010), p. 70 (DeFalco 2010).

[13] See, for example, Robert E. Yahnke, 'Old age and loss in feature-length films', *The Gerontologist*, 43 (2003), pp. 426–428 (Yahnke 2003), and Kurt Segers, 'Degenerative dementias and their medical care in the movies', *Alzheimer Disease and Associated Disorders*, 21 (2007), pp. 55–59 (Segers 2007).

[14] Eakin, *How Our Lives Become Stories*, p. 46 (Eakin 1999); Diedrich, *Treatments*, pp. 118, 142 (Diedrich 2007).

Confirming this general take on Bayley's trilogy, the German journalist Tilman Jens compares, amongst others, his father's need for close contact with Iris Murdoch's 'terror of being alone, of being cut off for even a few seconds from the familiar object' (96 in Bayley).[15] That Jens appropriates Bayley's metaphors may anticipate his feeling uncomfortable with his own picturing: while the British scholar presents us with a highly crafted illness memoir, organising it by the motif of Alzheimer's disease on the levels of story, text and narrative, Jens centrally speculates that his father's vascular dementia conveniently covered up his unwillingness to comment on his potential membership in the national-socialist party.

Against Michael Holroyd's ponderings on writing about his aunt, Tilman Jens's writing must seem highly unethical: it lacks any sensitivity in the context of discussing the father's past, which, unavoidably, contributes to the loss of the literary historian's reputation. These considerations become even more pressing in view of the fact that, as Claudia Mills has observed, the success of memoirs 'as a literary genre has sometimes been linked with a growing culture of narcissism'.[16] Indeed, the rage speaking from Gertrude Himmelfarb's commentary or A. N. Wilson's memoir reflects the heated atmosphere surrounding the publication of Bayley's texts at a time when his wife was still alive or her death still fresh (this judgement shifted for critics like Roger Lewis with the study of Murdoch's letters published in 2015).[17] Wilson, in particular, identified 'resentments, envy, poisonously strong misogyny and outright hatred of his wife' in Bayley's memoirs, and claimed that Bayley had publicly admitted that '[he has] never set much store by the truth'.[18] The philosopher Galen Strawson, by comparison, believed that

---

[15] Tilman Jens, *Demenz. Abschied von meinem Vater* [Dementia. Farewell to my father] (Gütersloh: Gütersloher Verlagshaus, 2009), p. 42 (T. Jens 2009); further references incorporated in the text.

[16] Claudia Mills, 'Friendship, fiction, and memoir: trust and betrayal in writing from one's own life', in *The Ethics of Life Writing*, ed. by Paul John Eakin (Ithaca: Cornell University Press, 2004), pp. 101–120, pp. 114, 111 (Mills 2004).

[17] Gertrude Himmelfarb, 'A man's own household his enemies', *Commentary Magazine*, 108 (1999), pp. 34–38, p. 35 (Himmelfarb 1999), and Richard Freadman, 'Decent and indecent: writing my father's life', in *The Ethics of Life Writing*, ed. by Eakin, pp. 121–146 (Freadman 2004); Roger Lewis, 'Oversexed, overpaid and underworked', *The Times*, 14 November 2015 (Lewis 2015).

[18] A. N. Wilson, *Iris Murdoch as I Knew Her* [2003] (London: Arrow Books, 2004), pp. 9, 257 (Wilson 2004).

'Bayley moves very close to truth' and saw a distinction between 'the whole truth' and the 'nothing-but-the-truth truth'.[19]

Strawson's perspective resonates with what psychoanalyst Donald Spence calls, and Arthur W. Frank refers to, as an exercise of narrative truth. By this, Spence means that the narrator attempts to re-establish the connection of past to present in the present of illness that was not planned in the past. This process does not involve the reinvention of the past, but 'the sense of what was foreground and background in past events can shift to recreate a past that displays [...] greater "continuity and closure"'.[20] This insight, in turn, is in line with our earlier observations of Bayley's search for continuity. Diedrich, who reads Bayley's memoir against Murdoch's philosophy, brings these moral considerations to the point, as she suspects that:

> Murdoch would view the proliferation of memoirs in contemporary culture with weariness at best, not necessarily because it is a popular, democratic rather than a high literary form, but because it is a form that often privileges the cultivation of a unified self.[21]

Tilman Jens's poetic choices, indeed, appear self-serving, and only add to the father's undignified presentation. He frequently selects verbs associated with a child's behaviour (like 'begging for a tranquilliser tablet' or 'having to obey'), without explicitly owning up to such comparison. This strategy, which is as evasive as it is systematic, enhances the reader's impression that the son forces the father into inescapable diminishment. What is more, Tilman Jens claims himself to be aware of the ethical implications associated with writing about a living family member, when confessing: 'Ich ertappe mich immer wieder, wie ich [...] meinen demenz-kranken Vater, statt ihn im Präsens leben zu lassen, ihn im Präteritum [...] einsarge' [I catch myself out again and again how I (...) bury my dementia afflicted father in the past tense (...), instead of letting him live in the present tense; 24]. However, he specifically uses the present tense when referring to the father's confrontation with his past

---

[19] Galen Strawson, 'Telling tales', *The Guardian*, 6 September 2003 (Strawson 2003); for a rounded summary of contemporary critical reception, see: Anne Rowe, 'Critical reception in England of *Iris: A Memoir of Iris Murdoch* by John Bayley', *Iris Murdoch Newsletter*, 13 (1999), pp. 9–10 (Rowe 1999).
[20] Frank, *Storyteller*, p. 61 (Frank 1995).
[21] Diedrich, *Treatments*, p. 140 (Diedrich 2007).

rather than to explore his continued activity within the illness. This strategy forces the reader to witness and judge the father personally. Reflected against Bayley's choices, this strategy becomes even more problematic: Bayley (and Gillies after him) uses the present tense to take us into the sense of despair pertaining to the day-to-day confrontation with Alzheimer's disease as such.[22]

This passivity enforcing presentation runs strongly counter to concepts of hegemonic masculinity and independence.[23] Furthermore, as males are usually identified with their legacy, Jens's rendering the father's condition as mental rather than bodily further enhances the reader's aversion.[24] This is particularly true, since the son's emphasis on the father's loss of intellectual abilities and agency deprives Walter Jens of his former social identity as a mind-defined philologist; it literally reduces him to a 'living dead'.[25] In this respect, the reception of Jens's narrative was very similar to Bayley's. But Bayley's writing is permeated by allusions to the shared history of matrimony. In fact, the gravity of Tilman Jens's presentational choices becomes even clearer when reading about Inge Jens's memories of the couple's 'ideal of a partnership'. In her autobiography, Walter Jens's wife particularly emphasises the need to be able to resort to a 'durch die Krankheit nicht zerstörbare Vergangenheit' [past indestructible by the illness] with her husband.[26]

In a second book, Jens claims that his intentions had been to write against the taboo of dementia.[27] He specifically compares himself to the medical journalist Sylvia Zacharias. Zacharias had reported on her famous father's memory loss in a book, whose publication was championed by the Hirnliga

---

[22] Zimmermann, 'Journeys', p. 387 (Zimmermann 2013b).

[23] James A. Smith et al., '"I've been independent for so damn long!": independence, masculinity and aging in a help seeking context', *Journal of Aging Studies*, 21 (2007), pp. 325–335 (Smith et al. 2007).

[24] Fine and Asch, 'Introduction: beyond pedestals' (Fine and Asch 1988).

[25] Gert Ueding, 'Tilman Jens begräbt den lebendigen Vater' [Tilman Jens buries the living father], *Die Welt*, 18 February 2009 (Ueding 2009).

[26] Inge Jens, *Unvollständige Erinnerungen* [Incomplete memories] (Reinbeck bei Hamburg: Rowohlt, 2009), pp. 287, 283 (I. Jens 2009).

[27] Tilman Jens, *Vatermord. Wider einen Generalverdacht* [Patricide. Against a general suspicion] (Gütersloh: Gütersloher Verlagshaus, 2010) (Jens 2010); the small number of German caregiver texts could support Jens's claim, but numbers are not higher in other non-English speaking European countries. The only truly German taboo I see is, given the dramatic historical context, the question of assisted suicide.

[Brain alliance], an organisation supporting Alzheimer's disease research.[28] But in doing so, Jens overlooks that Zacharias had written her report ten years earlier, when the societal awareness regarding Alzheimer's disease was much smaller than at his time of writing: compared to the 1990s, the number of mentions of 'Alzheimer' in the two largest German broadsheet newspapers, *Süddeutsche Zeitung* and *Frankfurter Allgemeine Zeitung*, tripled between 2000 and 2009. Moreover, the reader's preconception of males as preferring to act in a planned and rational manner will not facilitate Tilman Jens's efforts to encourage a more lenient judgement, especially, since a father–son relationship is often viewed as competitive.[29] In fact, it may be the sum of these impressions that led to Tilman Jens's work being set in the context of an alleged Oedipal relationship with his mother, not least since his dedication reads 'Für Mami' [for mommy].[30] Thinking in psychoanalytical terms, Tilman Jens's damaging narrative tactics could also be read as his inability to deal with the loss of the father as a powerful and allied figure. In any event, such controversial debate further removed both text and reader from the ostensibly intended discussion of dementia that already seemed a pretext rather than the purpose of Jens's writing.

Against these considerations, we would expect a son's account of his mother's Alzheimer's disease to be differently accentuated. The Canadian Jean Grothé chronicles his mother's illness in fourteen photographs and related short notes, literally presenting portraits of her, as she is passively seated in nine of these images.[31] Laying down the contrast between their

---

[28] Sylvia Zacharias, *Diagnose Alzheimer: Helmut Zacharias. Ein Bericht* [Diagnosis Alzheimer's: Helmut Zacharias. A report] (Cologne: Hirnliga e. V., 2000) (Zacharias 2000); 'Hirnliga e. V. – Deutschlands Alzheimer Forscher', http://www.hirnliga.de/index.html (accessed August 2016).

[29] Kory Floyd and Mark T. Morman, 'Human affection exchange: affectionate communication in father–son relationships', *The Journal of Social Psychology*, 143.5 (2003), pp. 599–612 (Floyd and Morman 2003); Karen L. Fingerman et al., 'Ambivalent relationship qualities between adults and their parents: implications for both parties' well-being', *The Journals of Gerontology, Series B: Psychological Sciences and Social Sciences*, 63.6 (2008), pp. P362–P371 (Fingerman et al. 2008).

[30] Iris Radisch, 'Der Mann seines Lebens. Tilman Jens verklärt und denunziert seinen an Demenz erkrankten wehrlosen Vater Walter Jens' [The Man of his life. Tilman Jens distorts and denounces his demented defenceless father Walter Jens], *Die Zeit*, 19 February 2009 (Radisch 2009).

[31] Jean Grothé, *Alzheimer. Un journal photographique* [Alzheimer's. A photographic diary] (Montreal: Les 400 coups, 2007) (Grothé 2007); references incorporated in the text.

former contentment and the life under the spell of Alzheimer's disease, the journal opens with a scene witnessing the life-long affectionate mother–son relationship: the mother wears an elegant dress, and, seated at the laid table of a restaurant opposite the photographer and son, directly focuses on Grothé; her charming smile signals full awareness of him and her being photographed (13).

I began a seminar on dementia pharmaceutical care using this photograph; the overwhelming student response described this take as depicting 'an elderly lady having lunch'. When I later showed a sequence of further photographs (17, 31, 33, 37), seminar attendants interpreted the less and less elegant dress and fashionable hairstyle, and the reduced eye contact as well as growing distance to the photographer as the photographer's way of documenting the lady's aging process; a process of decline and loss.[32]

The choice *and* reception of this portrayal bring home that Grothé equates dementia with aging and considers it a condition of loss and decline. Moreover, Grothé exposes his mother's frailty without any reservation. He reveals the precariousness of her condition in an again blurred photograph taken from an angle, which shows her as if on a sinking ship (25); depicts her on a hospital stretcher, following an ischemic attack that accelerates her decline (26); and shows her, dressed in a nightgown, in a dishevelled state (33). But even though the text completes this image of inescapable dissolution, Grothé's photographs provoke an ambiguous reading: he observes the mother's glum decline, but equally senses the hope in her continued identity within the illness.[33] Grothé achieves this effect by visually dissociating the illness from the person, as he continues to focus on the mother's gaze, while letting the surrounding objects and her shrinking body sharply determine her departure. Especially in the series of photographs I used for teaching, Grothé shows his mother on the impersonal settee (17), and later a chair of the nursing home (31), and, finally, two types of wheelchairs (33, 37).

The most telling photo is taken in a big white exhibition hall, in whose centre the small figure of the mother appears as a misplaced object without

---

[32] Zimmermann, 'Integrating medical humanities', p. 3 (Zimmermann 2013a).

[33] Ed Kashi's photographs reveal a similar ambiguity that embraces both the possibilities and limitations linked to aging, with their ambivalence being carried by their serving different societal or political connotations of aging; see: Carol Squiers, 'Ed Kashi. Aging in America', in *The Body at Risk. Photography of Disorder, Illness, and Healing* (Berkeley: University of California Press, 2005), pp. 192–209 (Squiers 2005).

relation to the surroundings, let alone the photographer (21). The distance between patient and photographer visualises the pair's mutual helplessness, especially as they are both exposed to the oppressive emptiness of the hall; the isolating consequences of the condition. The accompanying text reveals the core of this pain that explains Grothé's experience of loss in psychological terms: 'elle en vienne à fabuler, me prenant pour son mari. [...] Nous sommes revenus tous deux épuisés, peinés, troublés' [she begins to make up stories, taking me for her husband (...) we came back both of us exhausted, pained, disturbed; 20]. Aware that his mother is about to forget him, Grothé clings to the mother as perceiving of him as her son, continuing his documentation with a close-up portrait in which his mother clearly and lovingly focuses on him (23).

But considered from this perspective, this photographic series turns into a study on the eye contact a mother maintains with her son as a metaphor for a dementia patient's mental acuity. Consequently, we as onlookers – like the son and photographer – must wonder, and that more and more with every photograph, whether Mme Grothé continues to be cognitively aware; whether she continues to recognise her son, or whether her smile occurs in the reflex of having been a life-long age-old and now old age object of the son's camera. Grothé himself obviously ponders this question: he shows his mother as laughingly covering up her face, playfully peering through the slits formed by her fingers (19), while perceiving of her as 'jamais [...] si gamine auparavant' [never before (having been) so childlike; 18].

Grothé uses here a term that evokes notions of aging as a process of regression into a second childhood, with this understanding coming close to Tilman Jens's view of his father, and both explainable in psychoanalytical terms. But he links this expression to a photograph that takes in Mme Grothé's continued identity. In this way, Grothé signals, unlike Jens, that he keeps seeing his parent in the individual of changed behaviour and bodily appearance. In addition, the temporal immediacy conveyed in Grothé's photographs is less exposing than Jens's use of the present tense, because Grothé remains focused on the mother's presence as such, rather than the father's acts in the past. Indeed, Jens hardly lingers on the father's condition as one of aging, or decline in aging. Much rather, he emphasises the father's loss of agency.

That said, also Grothé's photographs transport concepts of mental confusion and passivity, and they picture dementia as a condition intricately linked to bodily decline. Having shown concern about how the film adaptation of Bayley's memoir presents embodiment, some critics might take issue with Grothé's work, because it reduces his mother to the body. Specifically in relation to Richard Eyre's *Iris*, Josephine Dolan and colleagues have asserted that:

> 'Iris' increasingly *becomes* her body as the Alzheimer's takes hold, no longer cerebral but physical. Murdoch's status as a highly intellectual writer is eroded by the image of her as an abject female body – and by the pathologization of that body as a site of mental and moral decline. The figure of the active, independent and fiercely intellectual younger woman is systematically replaced by that of the passive and dependent older one.[34]

That said, critics like Pia C. Kontos have viewed such a perspective on embodiment more positively, because it can further the viewer's empathy.[35] This interpretation perhaps furnishes an explanation for the engagement by students when I used Grothé's photographs in my teaching.

On the other hand, David Orr and Yugin Teo have, in negotiation with the work by Kontos and Dolan and colleagues, criticised the movie for foregrounding John Bayley's attempts to maintain Murdoch's selfhood as a writer.[36] Bayley's tendency to privilege the intellectual aspects of his wife's identity (despite perceiving of her as childlike) counters Jens's intellect-denying approach. Tilman Jens denies his father what I would like to term an extra-intellectual or, as Jens Brockmeier would say, pre-narrative identity. Grothé's photographs, by comparison, offer in their imagery per se such a pre-narrative identity, which, at its core, tells about the nurturing mother–son relationship. Concurrently, however, the presentation of portrait-like photographs neglects the fact that 'the displays of [the patient's] personality and character [...] require, for their very existence, interpersonal interaction and the social recognition given by others'.[37] We have seen such a recognition speaking from Judith Fox's presentation – an enormous

---

[34] Josephine Dolan, Suzy Gordon and Estella Tincknell, 'The post-feminist biopic: re-telling the past in *Iris*, *The Hours* and *Sylvia*', in *Adaptation in Contemporary Culture. Textual Infidelities*, ed. by Rachel Carroll (London: Continuum, 2009), pp. 174–185, p. 178 (emphasis original) (Dolan et al. 2009).

[35] Pia C. Kontos, 'Embodied selfhood in Alzheimer's disease. Rethinking person-centred care', *Dementia*, 4 (2005), pp. 553–570 (Kontos 2005).

[36] David M. R. Orr and Yugin Teo, 'Carers' responses to shifting identity in dementia in *Iris* and *Away From Her*: cultivating stability or embracing change?', *Medical Humanities*, 41 (2015), pp. 81–85 (Orr and Teo 2015).

[37] Sabat, *The Experience of Alzheimer's Disease*, p. 18 (Sabat 2001).

achievement if we take into account that Fox writes with the added pressure of caring for her husband, while also losing him to dementia.

In summary, the visual image of a patient relates the condition as embodied. Given that concepts of the aging process seemingly fit those of the disease trajectory, a patient's visual image may, therefore, quickly emerge as one of an elderly person. In addition, presentations of passivity and dependence in a female patient are perceived of as less ethically problematic because cultural concepts link being female by itself to such characteristics. On a second consideration, the core stigma attached to dementia, however, relates to it being perceived of as a condition of the mind. I suggest that this fact offers an explanation as to why, as G. Thomas Couser has observed in 'Memoir and (lack of) memory', the Alzheimer's narratives that achieve larger sales and reviewer recognition centre on male patients: the loss of the male mind appears more profound. Regardless of the patient's sex, though, the conceptualisation of patients losing their mind can easily turn them into passive beings without their own voice or continued personhood. It is such images, in particular, that will not enhance a positive attitude within society towards the ill – who are mostly, but not always, the elderly – and neither towards their condition and their need for empathetic and identity-affirming accompaniment on their journey.

Contrasting this viewpoint, I will now illustrate how two narrators rise above the disease-imposed temptation to objectify the patient's body, or to see their mind destroyed. Both Phillip Toledano and Arno Geiger follow the conviction expressed by psychiatrists and philosophers that patients 'should be treated as wholes'.[38] They perceive of dementia as an integral part of their parents' personality and natural aging.

Alzheimer's and Aging: The Patient as Subject

Phillip Toledano's text–photo composition opens with a portrayal of the father with a sunhat.[39] Mr Toledano looks absorbed in his world of thought; his gaze is directed downwards, but he demonstrates presence

---

[38] Hughes, Louw and Sabat, 'Seeing whole', p. 4 (Hughes et al. 2006).

[39] Phillip Toledano, *Days with My Father* (San Francisco: Chronicle Books, 2010) (Toledano 2010); some of the photographs referred to in the following can be seen on Phillip Toledano's webpage: 'Mr Toledano. *Days with My Father*', http://www.mrtoledano.com/days-with-my-father/01-Days-with-my-father (accessed August 2016).

and thoughtfulness; the hat gives him a look of independence and individuality. In this spirit, the son to an American father (an immigrant from Italy) and a French Moroccan mother shows – to follow Steven R. Sabat's definition – the father in his continuously lived, various social personae. In text and image, Toledano depicts him as the energetic storyteller, gesturing theatrically to illustrate his funny anecdote reported on the opposite page; the self-deprecating man, laughing and, with two pointedly shaped cookies on his chest, demanding the viewer to 'look at my titties!'; the emotional parent, in tears, affectionately embracing his daughter-in-law; the ailing patient, aware of his wife being dead and his memory fading, with his eyes closed, his cheeks sunken in, half his face in the shadow cast by himself.

Most of all, Toledano portrays his father as active agent of the story beyond his physical death. Mr Toledano's death makes the bereft son the object, as he is photographed in the pain of loss and separation. This scene strongly enhances the perception that Toledano preserves the father's dignity. The collection of photos is interspersed with records of the father's old age (a close-up of his wrinkly hand full of age spots; his exhausted face reaching out of the bath tub; his mouth agape while sleeping) that allude to his imminent death. His actual death, however, is documented in the son's tear-swollen gaze, directed diagonally downwards onto the opposite, white page that carries at its centre the text: 'My dad died yesterday'. As such, the question of ethicality regarding the patient's presentation comes down to how the reader works through the frequently blank pages that leave ample space for deliberations on the patient's mental state. It comes down to, as Rita Charon would say, 'the meaning [...] *created by* the meeting between teller and listener'.[40]

Like Fox, Toledano builds on the meaning of absence, as only one photo actually hints, in its blurredness, at the father's decreasing awareness. This choice strongly suggests that he considers, in comparison to Ernaux or Grothé, the parent's condition as neither constituting nor altering his personality. Consequentially, Toledano's work does not – unlike Grothé's photographs, which are sorted by date – chronicle decline: it represents an 'ongoing record of my father, and of our relationship. For whatever days we have left together'. The pages of his book are not numbered, as if to signal that the order of the photos could be changed, as they simply depict days spent with an individual, his character and

---

[40] Charon, *Narrative Medicine*, p. 52 (emphasis original) (Charon 2006).

identity – reminiscent of Konek's attempt to record the father in textual snippets. What is more, given that Toledano had been blogging his photos and experiences throughout these three years, his book authentically records the living time in both image and text.[41]

That such blogging seems more ethical than Mary Wilhoit's online diary, let alone Tilman Jens's depiction, is intricately linked to Toledano's reverential presentation of the father as continued parent outside the illness. I see such reverence particularly evident in images that echo personality traits like openness or extraversion that have been attributed to positive aging and suggested as supporting better coping with cognitive decline.[42] Toledano, for example, writes:

> My father had no time for old age. He was like a river. Always in motion, flowing forward with loose-limbed vigor. Sweeping past every obstacle with a smile, dancing and shimmering in the sun. Every door was there to be opened. Every window to be looked through.

Additionally, the accompanying photo depicts a flowery curtain in movement, suggesting that the 'river' will continue to flow behind this veil – in the reader's as well as the son's imagination. Such closure strongly underlines the father's autonomy and resonates with Fox's presentation of her husband that continues to speak to her as the loving wife. Grothé's portrayal, in contrast, does not leave any room for interpretation outside the mother's illness. This is particularly true, because her increasingly practical hairstyle and dreary clothes, when living in the nursing home, virtually trace her deterioration and anticipate her death. (As an aside, I used some of Toledano's photographs in the teaching session, in which I also used Grothé's series. Confronting students with these images triggered thoughtful and lively discussions on the caregiver's and patient's losses, and encouraged me to use illness life-writing more and more in

---

[41] The blog had previously been available on: http://www.huffingtonpost.com/phillip-toledano/fathers-day-is-days-with_b_617398.html, and: www.dayswithmyfather.com (both accessed December 2015); in such a blog, the sequence of photographs is, of course, a necessary given, but they lack the predetermining nature seen in Grothé's arrangement.

[42] Anne Boland and Philippe Cappeliez, 'Optimism and neuroticism as predictors of coping and adaptation in older women', *Personality and Individual Differences*, 22.6 (1997), pp. 909–919 (Boland and Cappeliez 1997); Robert Hill, *Positive Aging. A Guide for Mental Health Professionals and Consumers* (New York: W. W. Norton, 2005), pp. 96–118 (Hill 2005).

pharmaceutical care, in the conviction that it will also help reshape the general societal dementia narrative.)

The Austrian writer Arno Geiger, by comparison, rediscovers the father in his very illness experience.[43] This understanding is symbolised in the leitmotif of the father's photo, which the father had carried in his wallet since returning from the war, showing his wartime suffering. As this photo is now lost, Geiger realises, 'dass nicht nur das Foto auf einer Schutthalde gelandet war, sondern auch das Wissen, das mein Vater über seine Vergangenheit gehabt hatte' [that not only had the photo ended up on a rubbish dump, but so also had the knowledge that my father had about his past; 27]. As the father lost the photo, he loses his memory. As the son searches for this photo, he searches for the father's memory and the father himself. These efforts echo the urgency of other adult-child caregivers – I am particularly thinking of Konek or Ernaux – to counterbalance their parent's memory loss in the awareness of their insufficient knowledge, and the imminent ebbing of the parental source of knowledge, of the parent's past. Consequentially, Geiger places the finding of the photo in the centre of the narrative, when he describes the decision actively to take notes on the father's changes; these will become the basis of his documentation of the father's unbroken identity within dementia. This decision is reminiscent of Gillies's turn of mind, as she switches to writing down her experience of caregiving instead of pursuing the creation of a fictional story. Yet, her decision gains a different notion, since she admits to surrendering to the exhaustion of caregiving, while Geiger attempts to picture the father in his past and present life.[44]

Geiger portrays a father who continues to radiate warmth, wit and wisdom, the fruits of a lifetime: 'Er hatte seine Erinnerungen in Charakter umgemünzt, und der Charakter war ihm geblieben' [He had turned his memories into character, and this character remained with him; 73].[45] In this spirit, he interprets the father's condition as a continuation of his life-long search for security and belonging, after wartime

---

[43] Arno Geiger, *Der alte König in seinem Exil* [The old king in his exile] (Munich: Carl Hanser, 2011) (Geiger 2011); references incorporated in the text.
[44] Zimmermann, 'Journeys', p. 387 (Zimmermann 2013b).
[45] The dialectics of old age has been explored widely; see, e.g., Gerald F. Manning, 'Spinning the "globe of memory": metaphor, literature, and aging', pp. 37–55 (Manning 1991), and Warren A. S. Davidson, 'Metaphors of health and aging: geriatrics as metaphor', pp. 173–198 (Davidson 1991), both in *Metaphors of Aging in Science and the*

experiences of imprisonment and illness; hence, as a constituting and integral part of his aging, not like Ernaux as an enhancer of old age. In this respect, Geiger's approach reads like an implementation of Tom Kitwood's demands to see dementia as being determined by how health, biography and personality are constellated within the patient's life.[46] In fact, as Alzheimer's destroys the father's awareness of being at home, everything is now 'zerrüttet, der Mann, das Haus, die Welt' [destroyed, the man, the house, the world; 168]. This staccato zooms out from the individual afflicted by the disease to society that is subject to degeneration. It makes the perceived impact of Alzheimer's disease palpable, and recapitulates what Geiger states earlier:

> Alzheimer [ist] ein Sinnbild für den Zustand unserer Gesellschaft. Der Überblick ist verlorengegangen, das verfügbare Wissen nicht mehr überschaubar, pausenlose Neuerungen erzeugen Orientierungsprobleme und Zukunftsängste.
>
> [Alzheimer's (is) an allegory for the state of our society. The overview is lost, the knowledge available not manageable any more, constant innovation causes problems of disorientation and fear of the future; 58].

This point of view closely links the father's frailty and cognitive losses to his remaining world of experience, which is '[d]er einzig verbliebene Platz für ein Miteinander, das sich lohnte, [...] die Welt, wie der Vater sie wahrnahm' [the only remaining space for a worthwhile being together, (...) the world as perceived by the father; 117]. Geiger gives him his own narrative space: the twelve chapters are separated by sections printed in italics, whose length amounts to up to three pages. These sections reproduce snippets of dialogues between father and son in direct speech, so that the reader directly witnesses August Geiger's continued awareness, devoid of the son's interpretation.

This very strategy releases the patient from his 'exile' – his, to put it with Hawkins, 'estrangement, alienation, and separation' owing to

---

Humanities, ed. by Gary M. Kenyon, James E. Birren and Johannes J. F. Schroots (New York: Springer Publishing Company, 1991).

[46] Tom Kitwood, 'The dialectics of dementia: with particular reference to Alzheimer's disease', *Ageing and Society*, 10 (1999), pp. 177–196 (Kitwood 1999).

decreasing communication skills.⁴⁷ It makes him all the more 'king' of the narrative. In agreement with Jane Crisp's work, this narrative choice underlines Arno Geiger's perception that the patient's talking is a functional means for reconstructing his identity. Such living conversation is an even stronger testament to the patient's autonomy than Konek's descriptive considerations of her father's teaching, and it highlights the acute pain felt by caregivers like Reeve Lindbergh, whose parent stops speaking. This impression is reinforced by several formal differences in these narrative renderings: Konek's disruptive construction emphasises the need for continuity in her *own* outlook, while Geiger's decision to alternate chapters relating the father's past with those telling of current cognitive difficulties frames his view of the coherence maintained between the father's past personality and in his present illness. Gillies's choice to add disrupting chapters that relate socioscientific considerations regarding Alzheimer's disease, by comparison, emphasises the disruptive powers of the condition itself.⁴⁸

In line with these considerations, Arno Geiger's final chapter embodies continuity, as it presents the son's aphoristic deliberations on life, death and fate. Some of these are printed in italics, as if to indicate his learning from the father, with continuity being maintained and parenthood fulfilled. At the same time, this textual disruption visualises the son's struggle in view of his father's imminent death. In fact, Arno Geiger 'wollte über einen Lebenden schreiben, ich fand, dass der Vater, wie jeder Mensch, ein Schicksal verdient, das offenbleibt' [wanted to write about a living person, I believed that the father, like every human being, deserves a fate that remains open; 189]. This approach strongly furthers an understanding of Geiger's perception of his story not needing any enforced closure, whose focus would turn, as in Konek's, Ernaux's or Gillies's case, to the caregiver's survival. Likewise, this choice is evidence of Geiger's moral stance: it counter-narrates the reifying and infantilising conceptualisation of the patient – which led to his text being seen as a powerful counterstatement to Jens's publications.⁴⁹ At the same time, such open-endedness avoids writing about the most challenging aspects

---

⁴⁷ Hawkins, *Reconstructing Illness*, p. 79 (Hawkins 1999).

⁴⁸ Zimmermann, 'Journeys', p. 387 (Zimmermann 2013b).

⁴⁹ Birgit Nüchterlein, 'Zuhause ist jetzt anderswo' [At home is now elsewhere], *Nürnberger Nachrichten*, 16 February 2011 (Nüchterlein 2011).

of the illness experience: when the parent's loss of awareness and bodily disintegration leave little room for a narrative turn that would comply with the reader's desire for a positive closure.

Historical, Cultural and Personal Context Influence Attitudes to Dementia

Geiger's and Toledano's positive presentations may well be rooted in the men's upbringing in an environment that values the extended family – Geiger grew up in a remote village in the Austrian mountains, while Toledano was shaped by a Mediterranean, family-oriented education. This view is in tune with Woodward's considerations of Inoue's *Chronicle of My Mother*. Woodward identifies the influence of a less success-driven cultural context in the Japanese man's literary interpretation of his mother's Alzheimer's disease. In particular, she sees him focused 'on a literary rendering or interpretation of the disease rather than on clinical description of it', while Roach's mother merely serves as 'the vehicle for the subject of the essay'.[50]

In addition, both sons place their emphasis on aging as the final stage of life-long development. They come to see Alzheimer's disease as integral to aging, which strongly enables their patients and the reader's positive perception of them. Geiger's move to include his father's aphoristic musings is additionally enabling and resonates with Lindbergh's presentation of her mother. In fact, even though Lindbergh's mother is, like Grothé's mother, pictured as sitting on the settee most of the time, we gain the impression of a more rounded presentation of Anne Morrow Lindbergh. This is the case, because the daughter links her mother – in contrast to Tilman Jens's choices of presentation – to the history of her own work, quoting from her mother's poems and other writing at the beginning of almost every chapter of the memoir.

Grothé's and Jens's renderings of their respective parent is dominated by gender-related interpretations of Alzheimer's disease, which leads to passivity-suggesting portrayals. At the same time, the presentation and reception of John Bayley's writings highlight that the patient's life history strongly influences, perhaps even dictates, how the condition is

---

[50] Woodward, 'Reminiscence and the life review', pp. 139, 140 (Woodward 1986).

being perceived; in Iris Murdoch's like in Walter Jens's case as a loss of mind rather than an illness related to aging. Patient passivity is similarly seen in presentations that are, like Spohr's, embedded in, or conditioned by, the strain of caregiving. This onus, as we have seen, may be conducive to reducing the patient to a child, if not the object of the burden. What is more, given that the carer is frequently nursing a patient suffering from *later stages* of Alzheimer's disease (as in works by Ernaux or Konek), the adult child's or spouse's portrayal reflects the relative's *advanced* cognitive impairment and consequential need for guardianship. This constellation further takes away an understanding of the patient's continued autonomy and self.

We may certainly argue that, once his father was put into a nursing home, Geiger could write so positively, by adopting the perspective of 'care-free' distance, when 'eine Betreuung [zu Hause] auf diesem Niveau trotz intensiver Unterstützung durch die Familie nicht mehr möglich [war]' [caregiving at home on this level was not possible any more despite intensive support from the family; 134]. He is very much aware of the close interdependence between patient perception and quality of caregiving. This is why he appreciates, as I have discussed in relation to Reeve Lindbergh's presentation of her mother, true quality time with his father. Such quality time is very clearly dependent, as Geiger remarks, on the father's wellbeing:

> Was für eine Befreiung, wieder Lebensfreude zu spüren [...]. Jetzt [...] verfügte ich nicht nur über Zeit, sondern auch über Energie [... und der Vater war vom ersten Tag an ...] ausgeglichen, entspannt und aufmerksam.
>
> [What a relief to feel zest for life again (...). Now I did not only have time, but also energy and the father was equilibrated, relaxed and attentive from the first day on; 144–145].

I want to expand further on the importance of appreciating the patient's continued self and identity for her/his wellbeing as well as a positive caregiver–patient relationship by offering an analysis of a short piece of autobiographically inspired fiction.[51] Building on 'experiences of visiting his grandmother in a nursing home', the writer and director Josh

---

[51] Josh Appignanesi, *Ex Memoria. Some Memories Fade. Others Keep Returning* (Missing in Action Films Ltd., 2006) (Appignanesi 2006).

Appignanesi used 'some of [his grandmother's] life history and experiences' to create the character Eva. Concerned with 'how strange the world must have looked from [his grandmother's] viewpoint', Appignanesi challenges the viewer to deliberate on Eva's anxieties, social skills, emotional needs and coping strategies in the confrontation with her caregivers in a short film.[52]

For fifteen minutes, the camera focuses almost exclusively on Sarah Kestelman's Eva. Only the first two minutes (0:17–2:30) show Eva in her twenties (Natalie Press), waiting for somebody in a forest glade. Taking into account the film's clues – the sound of shouting voices, gunfire and a departing car in the distance – against general knowledge about the Second World War, the onlooker must assume that Eva takes these signs as evidence of the man she is waiting for being deported. With this opening scene etched in their mind, viewers then witness Eva's day in the nursing home. They are forced to scrutinise Eva's face, as she sits in her wheelchair, for almost thirty seconds, before their attention is distracted by life in the home evolving around her. Still, the camera remains on Eva's eye level; short- to medium-distance shots keep the onlooker fixed on the main character; and long takes collapse diegetic and discourse time into one, so that the viewer feels that she/he witnesses events in real time.[53]

Eva appears isolated in the scene's foreground, especially as her silence is set against the caregivers' and home visitors' bustling and clearly perceived conversations in the background and, later, loud and disruptive noise from medical equipment. Appignanesi continues to further the viewer's impression of Eva's isolation in a family visit scene (6:15–10:20). With over four minutes, it is the longest shot. Even though surrounded by close family – her daughter and two grandsons – Eva appears cut off: the relatives rush through the background, and, busying themselves outside Eva's perceptual field, leave time for only one extended eye contact (with the older grandson) that lasts thirty-six seconds (9:15–9:51).

According to Robert Edgar-Hunt and colleagues, 'short films tend to be character driven, it is the characters that progress the narrative'.[54] In fact, despite Eva's superficially perceived passivity, the viewer is acutely

---

[52] Appignanesi, *Ex Memoria*, DVD discussion leaflet, pp. 5, 13.

[53] Robert Edgar-Hunt, John Marland and Steven Rawle, *The Language of Film* (Lausanne: Ava Publishing S. A., 2010) (Edgar-Hunt et al. 2010).

[54] Ibid., p. 63 (Edgar-Hunt et al. 2010).

aware that she thinks and feels throughout, that her tightening of the grip around her shirt collar and breathing heavily suggest deep emotional turmoil. In familiarising us with Eva's past at the beginning of the film, Appignanesi compels us to read her behaviour and reactions to visual and auditory triggers – such as the voice of a German patient in the home, or the caregivers' pulling at her stockings and knickers as they want to help her go to the toilet – in the context of this initial scene and, thus, as building on Eva's memories. This presentation matches Jane Crisp's above-introduced view that added external information can elucidate the meaning of a patient's articulation. Likewise, it illustrates observations by The Bradford Dementia Group (who, together with the Wellcome Trust, supported the film's production) which suggest that patients relate what happens in the now of the care home environment to events in their past.[55]

When Eva escapes from her carers, the viewer becomes most acutely aware that her life history constitutes a major component of her present identity. Once caught and dragged back into her wheelchair, she asserts: 'you have the wrong one, the wrong one, you have the wrong one. It isn't me' (13:00). Reading these events in the light of her troubled past, the viewer must conclude that Eva continues to fear being deported herself, especially as she then implores the caregiver, who kneels down beside her wheelchair: 'you'll help me with my papers' (13:44). The caregiver, clearly uncomfortable with Eva offering 'anything you want, anything you want, right now' (13:52) in recognition of his anticipated administrative help, eventually mumbles that 'everything is in order' (14:08). While he cannot wholeheartedly enter into the conversation, his reaction mindfully responds to her emotional urgency, and relieves Eva greatly: her facial expression turns into a smile, as she raises her gaze upwards (14:40–14:58).

---

[55] Andrea Capstick, 'From room 21: narratives of liminality, shared space, and collective memory in dementia care', presentation at the conference 'A Narrative Future for Health Care', London, 20 June 2013; Capstick and colleagues capture 'the fragments and remains of the memories of people who have dementia' in the framework of the Trebus project; see: 'The Trebus Project', http://www.trebusprojects.org/ (accessed October 2016); see also: Robyn Westmacott et al., 'The contribution of autobiographical significance to semantic memory: evidence from Alzheimer's disease, semantic dementia, and amnesia', *Neuropsychologia*, 42.1 (2004), pp. 25–48 (Westmacott et al. 2004).

Eva's escape also lets us appreciate how well we actually can rely on her face, her mimics and gestures, for conversational clues. Eva disappears from the screen for an entire fifty-three seconds (12:03–12:56), while the camera's (and viewer's) gaze continues to focus on her empty wheelchair. During this interval, a bird comes to settle on its handle (12:27–12:45). Whether this bird metaphorically suggests Eva's freedom to fly during the time of her escape, or heightens the viewer's awareness of Eva's *person*hood being the anchor of information, is left to the viewer's interpretation. Such ambivalence purposefully fits with Appignanesi's core aim to 'encourage people to think about the uncomfortable issues raised by the film'.[56]

Aware that *Ex Memoria* may solicit strong reactions, the discussion guide takes up half of the DVD's information leaflet. It particularly includes guidelines for facilitating and structuring discussion and points to an additional 'learning package about dementia and care' online. This material covers topics such as 'dementia and communication', 'dementia and relationships' and 'what is person-centred care'.[57] Reading this list sheds further irony on the nursing home manager's assertion that 'the residents can spend their time how they like', while showing a visitor around (3:48). Eva is left alone with her emotional unrest, as none of the caregivers takes extended and loving note of her and her needs. This understanding is particularly troubling, since, in unison with the film's subtitle, *Some Memories Fade. Others Keep Returning*, the patient will continue to return to negotiating with her past – as suggested by the film's closing on a still image of the forest glade from the opening scene (14:58–15:09).

Considering the contrasting presentations explored and discussed in the two preceding chapters – some of them literally and metaphorically remove the patient's agency, others enable the patient as partner and independent storyteller – in the context of Appignanesi's portrayal of the

---

[56] Appignanesi, *Ex Memoria*, DVD discussion leaflet, p. 7. Also a recent collection of photographs that strictly focus on the faces of Alzheimer's patients leaves work to be done by the onlooker: the images are open to interpretation, confronting 'the observer with his or her own honesty, with his or her willingness to utilitarian compromises', as they may identify fear or 'radical honesty that speaks from these faces and eyes'; see: Peter Granser, *Alzheimer* (Heidelberg: Kehrer Verlag, 2008), preface, no page numbers (Granser 2008).

[57] www.exmemoriafilm.co.uk (accessed August 2013); the link is not accessible anymore upon redirection from: http://www.joshappignanesi.com/EX-MEMORIA (accessed August 2016).

patient's continued self, we are compelled to question the reliability of these accounts. This is also true, since caregivers frequently perceive of themselves as being sufferers in their own right: they try to locate themselves in their relative's memory loss and unstructured behaviour, and ask questions as to their own mortality and succumbing to the illness.

Ex Memoria makes us painfully aware of what it must feel like to be spoken about. Challenged to deliberate more fully on the individual's world of experience and perception by filmo-poetic renderings or photographic patient portrayals, we must move on to hearing patients' own accounts. This is also motivated by the fact that, as Vai Ramanathan puts it (and we have seen in Eva's case), remembering 'is not an individual process but a social one'.[58] In the following two chapters, I explore first-person accounts written by patients. Since writing, by itself and especially in the awareness of cognitive challenge, is already a sign of self-assertion, I particularly focus on how patients perceive of themselves within their condition and within such reifying and infantilising discourse.

---

[58] Ramanathan, *Alzheimer Discourse*, p. 29 (Ramanathan 1997).

Open Access This chapter is distributed under the terms of the Creative Commons Attribution 4.0 International License (http://creativecommons.org/licenses/by/4.0/), which permits use, duplication, adaptation, distribution and reproduction in any medium or format, as long as you give appropriate credit to the original author(s) and the source, a link is provided to the Creative Commons license and any changes made are indicated.

The images or other third party material in this chapter are included in the work's Creative Commons license, unless indicated otherwise in the credit line; if such material is not included in the work's Creative Commons license and the respective action is not permitted by statutory regulation, users will need to obtain permission from the license holder to duplicate, adapt or reproduce the material.

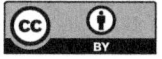

CHAPTER 4

About Tradition and Triumph: Patients Popularise Dementia Narrative

Abstract This chapter dissects how societal expectations regarding the dementia patient's performance and productivity impose successful narrative articulation as central to the perception of identity, social assertion and self. It explores the phenomenon that the first patient accounts present linear and edited (rather than chaos) narratives, and aims at understanding how the discrepancy between illness process and narrative plot impacts on the reader's perception of patient and condition. A comparison of patient- versus co-authored texts that additionally accounts for different stages in the severity of dementia is as revealing as an analysis of sequential publications by the same patient. This investigation supports the argument that gradually intensifying patient activism, also related to their popularising dementia narratives, enables patients' freedom of presentation towards structurally less accomplished accounts.

Keywords Articulacy · Illness description · Fragmented account · Linear narrative · Temporal coherence

> *The 36-hour Day* was about the best one I read. There was a lot of good information there, but it was mostly for caregivers. I could not see where any of it applied to me. I am just not like most of the Alzheimer's patients I read about. I can still think, talk, walk, write and do almost anything I want.[1]

> The fullness of who I once was will be seen in the simplicity of who I am within, surrounded by layer upon layer of memories.[2]

In 1998, Lawrence Cohen identified the practical knowledge of Alzheimer's disease in the American and Western European context to be organised around two manoeuvres:

> First, it involves an *iteration* of its pathology as opposed to its normality, despite the lack of a cure. Second, it involves a *circulation*: of legitimate suffering, between diseased and care-giving bodies.

Cohen notes an 'exchange of symptoms – the body of the caretaker for the body of the Alzheimer's patient', and observes how families were seen as being victimised by patients and their care.[3] Moreover, he argued that the general public appreciated a patient's personhood and subjectivity only in her/his choice to alleviate the caregiver's (in Cohen's phraseology, the caretaker's) burden. To illustrate his point, the ethnographer specifically referred to the 'voice' and 'action' of the patient Janet Adkins, who in 1990 ended her life with the help of the euthanasia activist Jack Kevorkian – a case that was broadly covered by the media.[4]

Cohen undertook his field research in India in the decade between 1985 and 1995, when patient life-writing was still in its infancy. From the vantage point of two decades' distance, the phenomena of exchange and circulation are perhaps most tangibly reflected in the numeric imbalance between caregiver and patient narratives from the condition's earliest appearance in book-length accounts: the patient is the told-about entity of care. This perspective is in line with John Wiltshire's particular

---

[1] Larry Rose, *Show Me the Way to Go Home* (Forest Knolls: Elder Books, 1996), p. 26 (manual title *sic*) (Rose 1996).

[2] Christine Boden, *Who Will I Be When I Die?* (Sydney: Harper Collins, 1998), p. 49 (Boden 1998).

[3] Cohen, *No Aging in India*, pp. 49, 51, 58 (emphases original) (Cohen 1999).

[4] See, for example, Timothy Egan, '"Her mind was everything," dead woman's husband says', *New York Times*, 6 June 1990 (Egan 1990).

emphasis on dementia as disrupting the pathographer's meaning of life, which he developed, in the year 2000, against an aesthetic analysis of two narratives that take the caregiver's point of view.

With Appignanesi's portrayal in mind, I argue that no narrative will embody Wiltshire's discernment relating to identity more directly than the dementia patient's *personal* account. If society in general – as much as policymakers, health-economists and medical practitioners – were to continue to overlook the patient, the perception of dementia and its bearing on identity would remain utterly limited and partial. This is especially true in the light of the advocacy speaking from both Larry Rose's and Christine Boden's statements, and insights gained from an analysis of interactional processes in patient narratives: 'AD patients, like those of us who are normal, are sensitive to audience, setting, topic, time, and so forth'.[5]

In other words, patients may well present and organise their life story with a specific agenda in mind. Consideration of patient-authored texts will significantly contribute to an understanding of the patients' attitude towards their condition and precarious identity. Moreover, it will enhance a discussion of how to adapt healthcare policies to changing demographic requirements. In this and the following chapter, I will introduce the few patient narratives that have been published in book format since 1989. Their perspective supplements the medico-scientific and healthcare discourses that continue to inform caregiver perceptions. It also provides direct action points for the development of a more patient-centred approach to caregiving.

My discussion of caregiver life-writing has revealed significant changes in patient representation over a thirty-year period. The discussion of patient narratives here is similarly organised according to their publication date. This approach will allow for a closer scrutiny of how patients' presentations negotiate with the slowly changing mainstream dementia narrative. This insight will further an understanding of the power and pressure lying in the societal conceptualisation of dementia and the healing effect an open acceptance and discussion of dementia can have – not only on the caregiver as we have seen above, but especially, and in the first place, on the patient.

The present chapter looks at patient narratives that emerged up to the early 2000s, during a period that saw, as Cohen would have it, caregivers

---

[5] Ramanathan, *Alzheimer Discourse*, p. 70 (Ramanathan 1997).

as secondarily victimised. It is in this atmosphere, I so argue in my analysis of the accounts by Robert Davis, Diana Friel McGowin and Larry Rose, that patients follow traditional narrative concepts. In agreement with early criticism of these narratives, I identify them as deploying linear plots and established myths.[6] But reading them from the vantage point of greater temporal distance, and in the context of Hawkins's illness narrative criticism as well as Couser's ethical considerations, I believe these authorial choices to be purposeful for the patients' wider political cause. At the time of publication, these narratives appealed to a readership primed for the caregiver's accomplished account. Complying with their readers' expectations, patients could begin to gather an audience that learned to appreciate the patient's continued personhood. It is against this changing background that slightly later published narratives could attempt a presentation that reflects the patient's narrative capabilities more credibly. My comparison of Cary Smith Henderson's narrative fragments to Thomas DeBaggio's highly articulate and literary composition illustrates how patients struggled to find narrative forms that would embrace the plot of their disease, while leaving space and scope for continued identity and personhood within this trajectory.

I close this chapter with an analysis of the account of a Harvard cardiologist about his Parkinson's disease with rapidly progressing Lewy body dementia. Building on life-long experiences from the vantage point of a practicing clinician, Thomas Graboys now takes the viewpoint of the patient. His change in perspective enables him to bring the patient's agenda to an audience that authoritatively includes the medical profession. Several years into patient life-writing, this agenda now can move on from the recovery of identity and personhood directly to address matters such as end-of-life treatment and choices.

TRADITION SELLS: THE JOURNEY INTO DARKNESS

The first patients reflecting on their Alzheimer's experience in book-length narratives report on *My Journey into Alzheimer's Disease*, describe their *Personal Journey through the Maze of Alzheimer's*, or demand to

---

[6] Basting, 'Looking back from loss' (Basting 2003); Ballenger, *Self, Senility, and Alzheimer's Disease*, esp. Chap. 6 (Ballenger 2006); Burke, 'Alzheimer's disease' (Burke 2007).

Show Me the Way to Go Home.[7] Taken as such, these patients picture their illness experience as a journey, which, in Arthur W. Frank's understanding, is 'a passage through real and symbolic dangers in preparation for the opportunity of a life enhanced by that passage'.[8] In her book on pathographies, Anne Hunsaker Hawkins illustrates that formulation (like the journey myth) gathers:

> together the separate meanings, the moments of illumination and understanding, the cycles of hope and despair, and weaves them into a whole fabric, one wherein a temporal sequence of events takes on narrative form.[9]

However, the degenerative chronicity of Alzheimer's disease necessarily prevents patients from truly returning from their illness experience, in terms of remission or healing. Therefore, the question is: how do these patients actually formulate their journey?

Robert Davis, vicar of one of Miami's largest churches, faces the harsh end of his career in his early fifties. Like Konek, Grothé and Geiger, he juxtaposes past to present, specifically telling readers in some detail about his childhood and his coming to Christ. In this way, he enhances the reader's understanding of how, in his illness, '[t]his personal and tender relationship that I had with the Lord was no longer there' (47). He uses imagery of sunlight to describe himself as living in the enlightened service of Christ. Images of darkness and an illustration of himself as 'sink[ing] more and more into the moonlight' (81), in turn, depict the contrast between his former life and the disease-enforced biographical disruption on a metaphorical level. In this context note how the world of experience behind notions of darkness and moon as compared to light and sun links to the concept of orientational metaphors, as illustrated by Lakoff and Johnson: light and brightness are linked to health and life, with the brightness itself alluding to the metaphoric illumination of the

---

[7] Davis, *My Journey into Alzheimer's Disease* (Davis 1989); McGowin, *Living in the Labyrinth* (McGowin 1993); Rose, *Show Me the Way to Go Home* (Rose 1996); references incorporated in the text.

[8] Arthur W. Frank, *At the Will of the Body. Reflections on Illness* (Boston: Mariner Books, 2002), p. 131 (Frank 2002); for a discussion of the 'quest narrative', see: Frank, *Storyteller*, pp. 115–136 (Frank 1995); on the journey myth in these 'conventional autobiographies', see also: Ballenger, *Self, Senility, and Alzheimer's Disease*, pp. 174–176 (Ballenger 2006).

[9] Hawkins, *Reconstructing Illness*, p. 24 (Hawkins 1999).

mind; darkness identifies with concepts of downward orientation and, thus, decline, sickness and death.[10] For the vicar, these images convey the full incredulity of his situation.

Davis opens his account with the passivity depicting metaphor of being a 'victim' (18), which strongly resembles Spohr's helpless verdict image, and resonates with Larry Rose's imagery that underlines his perception of helpless innocence. Specifically, Rose describes his initial confrontation with memory loss as feeling:

> the uncertainty of a person experiencing a hurricane or a tornado for the first time; the terrifying sensation that comes on realizing that what should be firm and solid is no longer so, and cannot be relied upon. (4)

Yet, Davis quickly moves on to interpret his illness as a godsend. In obedient acceptance, he sees his life turned 'from moonlight to sonlight' (129), when he comes to understand that:

> instead of my reaching out to Christ by prayer, intellectual determination, sheer bull-headed faith, or by aggressively claiming the promises of Scripture, Christ reached down and held me close to him [...]. From now on, my lot in life would be to be especially held by the Shepherd, letting him fully care for me. (55–56)

In this way, Davis is able to accept his expected chronic decline as a further lesson to learn 'the pure simple faith of a little child' (130), creating continuity between his life before and in the illness. Both fit into his biography of 'servanthood' (23). Similarly, Larry Rose maintains continuity by aiming to follow what his son's introduction to his narrative describes as his motto, namely never to:

> indulge in worry or self-pity. It will tear down your personality and destroy your skills. The only thing that will make any situation work is the attitude you develop toward it. (viii)

Indeed, Rose's publishing a further narrative in his more advanced condition, as well as his involvement in the Dementia Advocacy and

---

[10] Lakoff and Johnson, *Metaphors We Live by*, pp. 14–21 (Lakoff and Johnson 2003).

Support Network International (DASNI) additionally witness to his resilience.[11]

This very conceptualisation of continuity enables Davis to interpret disease-caused behavioural changes as furthering his spiritual life. In addition, it avoids disabling connotations of the medico-scientifically bolstered child metaphor that depict Walter Jens's exposedness or Hank Spohr's dependence. Taken together, Robert Davis's story follows the rites of passage that Hawkins identifies as core constituents of the patient's journey. Specifically, Davis's separation from his former life as a pastor is followed by a phase of learning, which, eventually, leads to his incorporating the condition into his life-long vocation as that of a strong Christian believer. Charles Schneider takes similar comfort in his Christian faith but pictures Alzheimer's as 'beast' and 'intruder', which suggests more ambivalent feelings.[12]

Likewise, Diana Friel McGowin takes us from initial memory lapses at the beginning of her 'unplanned journey' (1), through to her 'early retirement' (64), at the age of forty-five. She places this fact in the centre of her text to emphasise her concern about losing her identity as an accomplished legal secretary.[13] McGowin has enormous difficulty in accepting her condition:

> I recoiled in alarm at each additional loss of memory, and concentration. But I would not confide in family members as each additional loss occured. Instead I continued playing a camouflage game of 'I've Got a Secret', long after everyone knew. (97)

Following this initial phase of denial, she begins to articulate, as Basting puts it, 'the contradiction between her own feelings of self-worth and the depletion of her cultural value as a victim of Alzheimer's':

---

[11] Larry Rose, *Larry's Way. Another Look at Alzheimer's from the Inside* (Lincoln: iUniverse, 2003) (Rose 2003); 'DASNI annual general meeting 17 April 2003 – minutes', http://www.dasninternational.org/2003/2003agm_minutes.php (accessed August 2016).

[12] Charles Schneider, *Don't Bury Me, It Ain't Over Yet!* (Bloomington: Author House, 2006), pp. 4, 5 (Schneider 2006).

[13] The patient Tracy Mobley admits similar fears, in *Young Hope. The Broken Road* (Denver: Outskirts Press, 2007) (Mobley 2007).

If I am no longer a woman, why do I still feel I'm one? If no longer worth holding, why do I crave it? If no longer sensual, why do I still enjoy the soft texture of satin and silk against my skin? If no longer sensitive, why do moving song lyrics strike a responsive chord in me? My every molecule seems to scream out that I do, indeed, exist, and that existence must be valued by someone! (114)[14]

In time, McGowin refocuses her energies on her remaining abilities. Such shifting notions and rites of passage echo the stages of grieving that Elisabeth Kübler-Ross had identified for the process of mourning. This sequence is certainly transferable to the emotional upset resulting from McGowin's confrontation with memory loss.[15] But, especially in the light of patients' own assertions, I deliberately refrain from the self-suggesting comparison of 'death' to 'loss of self'. Confirming this perspective, McGowin energetically initiates the first patient-centred support group in her hometown Orlando, setting off a quickly spreading, nationwide movement that propagated patients' self-assertion.[16]

Nonetheless, the demonstration of such animated eloquence within a coherent narrative furthers the reader's inclination to view Davis, Rose or McGowin as fully able persons rather than cognitively challenged Alzheimer's patients. This is particularly true, since their erosion of memory allegedly places them beyond meaningful personhood, as has been claimed by social as well as clinical scientists.[17] However, these patients are all in stages of the condition that still allow them to perceive of the implications of their individuation being undone through their lack of narrative ability.[18] This very awareness leads them to 'describe' rather than

---

[14] Basting, 'Looking back from loss', p. 90 (Basting 2003).

[15] See also: Valerie Brandon, 'Foreword' to Jeanne L. Lee, *Just Love Me. My Life Turned Upside-Down by Alzheimer's* (West Lafayette: Purdue University Press, 2003), pp. xiv–xv, p. xv (Brandon 2003); on the relevance to the caregiver's experience of Kübler-Ross's stage model of dying, see: Gubrium, 'Narrative practice', pp. 195–198 (Gubrium 2000).

[16] Meg Grant, 'Looking into her labyrinth', *People*, 22 March 1993 (Grant 1993).

[17] See, for example, Andrea Fontana and Ronald W. Smith, 'Alzheimer's disease victims: the "unbecoming" of self and the normalization of competence', *Sociological Perspectives*, 32 (1989), pp. 35–46 (Fontana and Smith 1989); see also: Burke, 'Alzheimer's disease' (Burke 2007).

[18] On the intricate link between narrative and identity, and patients' writing against the historical background of the disciplinary use of diagnosis, i.e., their diagnosis-enforced

'perform' their condition, with the help of their acknowledged partners, and choose self-saving metaphors like the maze.[19] Davis publishes 'with help from his wife, Betty' (3), and McGowin closes with an epilogue 'by Diana McGowin & Jack McGowin' (117).

I see these considerations confirmed, when looking into Larry Rose's second text, published eleven years into his diagnosis. In this narrative, frequent typos witness disease progression. The same is true for his emphasis on significance rather than temporal sequence in chapters that reflect short attention span, as they hardly extend over more than two to three pages. Notably, *Larry's Way* has always only been available as print-on-demand – as are several other patient narratives I am referring to in this discussion. This fact tellingly discloses the publisher's concern that the story's lack of coherence would not make it a big seller, and it confirms that coherent narration contributes to the construction of a societally more valued self, on a personal and public level.[20]

Nevertheless, some texts perform the condition-enforced limits of expression, particularly in more advanced stages of the illness, while still serving the patient's agenda. Yet, I believe that such choices strongly rely on the first dementia patients, who stepped out of the shadow, to assert themselves in the public eye. Only once their identity was reclaimed in narrative forms accessible to the general reader, could more fragmented narration be accepted and published.

Form and Contents: Narrating Alzheimer's versus 'Account-Ability'

Cary Smith Henderson could not complete his book independently, since 'he still lives, but only in the sense of a beating heart and lungs that continue to take in air', as his wife informs us in the introduction to her husband's narrative.[21] The book's subtitle, *An Alzheimer's Journal*,

---

transformation into 'demented' subjects, see: Eakin, *Living Autobiographically*, p. 45 (Eakin 2008); Eakin particularly refers to Michel Foucault's work; see also: Ballenger, *Self, Senility, and Alzheimer's Disease*, p. 183 (Ballenger 2006).

[19] Basting, 'Looking back from loss', pp. 89, 92 (Basting 2003).

[20] Ryan, Bannister and Anas, 'The dementia narrative' (Ryan et al. 2009).

[21] Henderson, *Partial View*, p. xvii (Henderson 1998); further references incorporated in the text.

already suggests that its narrative form does not follow what we consider a classical autobiography. Henderson used a tape recorder to collect his moment-in-time thoughts and feelings over one year of his living with Alzheimer's. His daughter, later, transcribed his recordings in their original, disoriented structurelessness that we strongly witness in Henderson's inability to locate himself in time; Basting reads this as reflecting Henderson's lacking 'sense of beginning, middle, or end' in his journal:

> No two days and no two moments are the same. [...] I have no sense of time. [...] it may be just a short time that she's been away – it feels like forever [...]. It's just some kind of time warp. (47)[22]

Equally, we behold the repetitive nature of his musings that mainly centre around deprivation and loss, as 'Alzheimer's is [...] a maimer. I'm sure, a maimer of – what did I say? – certainly a killer of people's thoughts' (59).

The very repetitiveness of Henderson's fragments is the narrative performance of compulsiveness and short attention spans that Arthur W. Frank conceptualises as 'chaos narrative'. As I emphasised in the introduction, Frank's original description relates to caregiver accounts that evoke similarities with Ernaux's unstructured fragments. However, in my view, that his remarks perfectly match the patient's narrative performance tellingly highlights that patients can, indeed, narrate their fractured self.

As such, we come to appreciate the full picture of Henderson's different social selves, which Phillip Toledano so effectively depicts for his father, only in conjunction with his wife's introduction to the book. This introduction relates Henderson's characteristics as husband and history professor. Henderson, in turn, perceives of himself as a 'very second-class citizen in the real sense of the word' (74), but still sees himself as an 'onlooker and philosopher' (74). This very much suggests his continued sense of self-worth and desire to act, as also observed by Basting in relation to Henderson's participating in a drug study. About this contribution, Henderson feels:

> I'm doing something not only interesting but I think something that's needed [... which] makes me feel very good [...]. It makes me feel like I'm not going to just rot in my old age, helpless and stupid (63).[23]

---

[22] Basting, 'Looking back from loss', p. 95 (Basting 2003).
[23] Ibid. (Basting 2003).

I even believe that we appreciate Henderson as a *dependable* 'onlooker', since his deliberations strongly resonate with Susan Sontag's conceptualisation of the 'kingdom of the sick'.[24] His comment reveals Henderson's clear awareness of his precarious state and alerts the reader to the negative impact of the frequently disabling, since passive, patient conceptualisation perceived in the accounts of, for example, Betty Baker Spohr or Tilman Jens.

Despite being the author of the book in this precarious state, Henderson must become its object, when his wife reports on him and his daughter brings to life his recordings. I contend that this combination is necessary to make it a readable and sellable book that conforms to the Western achievermentality and offers a not too frightening image of the patient and his condition.[25] This understanding then is in line with Kathlyn Conway's remark – with reference to Frank's 'chaos narrative' – that:

> Without a speaker or writer to transform the experience into something coherent enough to be communicated, we are left, ironically, with a verbal chaos that fails to communicate the feel of chaos.[26]

The fact that the book is interspersed with photographs depicting Henderson in his condition, adds to the reader's perception of Henderson's limited ability and objectified performance – even though 'he chose to let me photograph him in order to share his life with others' (99), as the photographer Nancy Andrews acknowledges. Such a reading is supported by Jesse F. Ballenger's interpretation of these photos as depicting 'Henderson contending bravely in a world in which everyday objects became strange and threatening'; and Lucy Burke's observation that Henderson never 'engages eye contact directly with the camera'.[27] This latter fact sets our perception of Henderson apart from Judith Fox's

---

[24] Susan Sontag, *Illness as Metaphor* [1977] and *AIDS and Its Metaphors* [1988] (London: Penguin, 2002), p. 3 (Sontag 2002).

[25] Emily C. Bartels, 'Outside the box: surviving survival', *Literature and Medicine*, 28.2 (2009), pp. 237–252 (Bartels 2009); possibly, reduced pressure to perform explains the lack of dementia patient autobiographies in Europe as compared to the US.

[26] Conway, *Limits of Expression*, p. 105 (Conway 2007).

[27] Ballenger, *Self, Senility and Alzheimer's Disease*, p. 179 (Ballenger 2006); Burke, 'Alzheimer's disease', p. 12 (Burke 2007).

husband, Phillip Toledano's father, or even Jean Grothé's mother, whose gaze the son deliberately tries to catch and hold.

Against these considerations, the journal's title, *Partial View*, reflects Henderson's narrative limits. I even suggest that the reader's perception of Henderson's helpless disorientation comes closest to the less enabling patient presentations drawn by some caregivers. At the same time, however, it is exactly this limited ability to perform to society's expectations of an articulate social being that gives Henderson's reader the 'full view' of the adversities faced in the advanced stages of Alzheimer's disease. Because we begin, speaking with Hughes, Louw and Sabat, to see 'the person as a situated human being, who engages with the world in a mental and bodily way in agent-like activities'.[28]

Henderson's book, praised as an important contribution 'in its refusal to submerge difference and in its avowedly collaborative nature', clearly demonstrates that the reality of Alzheimer's disease goes beyond its clinical diagnosis and general societal perception.[29] It was published at a time, when the societal awareness of the condition began to increase, against the background of the Alzheimer's Association changing from being a group of passionate volunteers to becoming a professional organisation.[30] Thomas DeBaggio's narratives testify to the patient's perceived and performed individuality.[31] The journalist and herb grower writes in anticipation of losing his agency and independence, eventually even his dignity, musing to have 'only a few years before I become a hatstand' (58), and later on seeing himself 'rattl[ing] my cage but no one comes to feed me' (185). He uses metaphors that strip him of his humanity and personhood, and reduce him to an animal, even an inanimate object.

In addition, as I illustrate elsewhere, he employs highly charged images relating to death and dying, frequently referring to his 'death sentence' (1), and the disease process as 'biological war' (169) and 'holocaust of my brain' (184). In this way, he alludes to the impossibility

---

[28] Hughes, Louw and Sabat, 'Seeing whole', p. 35 (see above p. 11) (Hughes et al. 2006).
[29] Burke, 'Alzheimer's disease', p. 14 (Burke 2007).
[30] Basting, *Forget Memory*, p. 146 (Basting 2009); consider also therein Basting's useful 'timeline of stories and events in the recent history of dementia', pp. 181–186.
[31] Thomas DeBaggio, *Losing My Mind. An Intimate Look at Life with Alzheimer's* (New York: The Free Press, 2002) (DeBaggio 2002); references incorporated in the text.

of understanding the remorseless dying of brain cells and of expressing the pain experienced of imminent, relentless loss of self and life. This depiction highlights how cellular loss comes to make loss the all-encompassing medico-scientific metonym for perceived Alzheimer's disease-related changes. Elaine Scarry classifies biological war and holocaust as torture, and expands on how such experiences lie beyond the victim's verbalisation abilities. This perspective underscores, all the more, DeBaggio's speechlessness at the perceived atrocity of his diagnosis.[32] Reflecting Lawrence Cohen's perspective, the use of the victim metaphor illuminates how strongly *both* caregivers (think about Spohr's use of the victim image) *and* patients perceive of the passifying nature of the condition. DeBaggio's imagery pushes this understanding further towards notions of torture from within.

At the same time, DeBaggio claims to 'stumble through my shrinking vocabulary' (187), but later writes that: 'The childhood wounds healed, and my dreams were less haunted by fear. Imagination soon replaced anxiety and I learned early its lonely, lovely powers' (193). This section, in combining personification, image and enallage with alliterated rhyme and lyrically inspired word order, testifies to DeBaggio's exceedingly articulate style. In fact, as if directly following Scarry's insights into the making power of art in the face of illness, DeBaggio presents a thoughtfully crafted narrative that 'attempt[s] to show the parameters of long- and short-term memory and how Alzheimer's works to destroy the present and the past [... in] three narrative lines' (xi). These strands encompass his autobiography, quotations from scientific papers, and carefully constructed aphorisms, highlighted in italics. The latter sections bring out generalised fears surrounding his diagnosis, and are purposefully confirmed by the flash-forwards achieved with the scientific material.

Such astute textual representation led to his book quickly being interpreted as much more than the narrative of someone, who is 'writing in a panic' (25): clinical scientists doubted that DeBaggio was actually afflicted by Alzheimer's disease.[33] However, research shows that patients in early

---

[32] Scarry, *The Body in Pain* (Scarry 1985); Zimmermann, 'Alzheimer's disease metaphors' (Zimmermann forthcoming).

[33] Peter J. Whitehouse, 'Losing my mind. An intimate look at life with Alzheimer's', *New England Journal of Medicine*, 347.11 (2002), p. 861 (Whitehouse 2002); see also: Ballenger, *Self, Senility, and Alzheimer's Disease*, p. 227 fn. 54 (Ballenger 2006).

stages of the condition do retain figurative language.[34] In this awareness, and in my intentions to reflect on DeBaggio's narrative articulation in the context of the previously presented accounts, I believe, in comparison to Peter J. Whitehouse's objections, DeBaggio's purpose for writing to be more nuanced.

For DeBaggio, who harbours life-long regrets for having given up professional journalism, losing his ability to perform on a high linguistic level equals death. Writing in itself amounts to his holding on to his identity as a healthy human being, which, in turn, makes writing about his entire life a necessity. Living out his eloquence in the earliest days of his diagnosis is his way of giving meaning to his illness. He seizes the opportunity of 'finally [having] a story of hell to tell' (1), in which his poignant articulateness runs counter to the anticipated loss of acuity and agency, and provides the means to overcome imminent memory deficits. His text becomes immediate note-taking and his story the legacy for others.

This view is supported by looking at DeBaggio's second narrative.[35] Here, his metaphors pertain to the field of his long-lived profession as gardener, and picture events in his more advanced condition. Such observation is in agreement with research suggesting that Alzheimer's patients show low performance in novel metaphor comprehension.[36] Illustrating the brittleness of a tree in his garden, he 'remembered the long, fruitful life of the tree and the way its rich, hard essence returns to the earth as nourishment and provides new promise'. Given that the tree is generally perceived as a metaphor for the circle of life, DeBaggio seemingly hints at his own decreasing abilities. When then continuing with '[t]hus does the wealth of a single tree outlive the human memory and become timeless' (151), he pictures his helpless pain and loss: the actually inanimate object outlives the patient's powers.

Equally, DeBaggio explicitly acknowledges his family's strong input in composing especially this second narrative. While still serving different narrative strands, he fails to relate events on a coherent timeline

---

[34] Costanza Papagno, 'Comprehension of metaphors and idioms in patients with Alzheimer's disease', *Brain*, 124 (2001), pp. 1450–1460 (Papagno 2001).

[35] Thomas DeBaggio, *When it Gets Dark. An Enlightened Reflection on Life with Alzheimer's* (New York: The Free Press, 2003) (DeBaggio 2003); references incorporated in the text.

[36] Martina Amanzio et al., 'Metaphor comprehension in Alzheimer's disease: novelty matters', *Brain and Language*, 107 (2008), pp. 1–10 (Amanzio et al. 2008).

(ruminating instead over his professional backyard gardening), demonstrates memory loss (variously repeating himself) and reveals decreasing attention, as coherent sections become shorter. These very sections describe an elderly man in the third person, just as Konek chooses to depict her father's disappearance, as if DeBaggio was desperately picturing himself as he cannot be much longer. In particular, he closes on the note that 'the walker comes to a turning point, he adjusts his cap low on his head, preparing to look into the bright rising sun' (226). This image runs counter to the sunset that readers would expect, in view of the illness's prognosis as well as the narrative's aesthetic indications of decline. It underlines the author-narrator's need for positive closure in an unspeakable situation. At the same time, it becomes painfully ironic, when read against DeBaggio's death in February 2011.[37]

With Henderson's fragmented presentation in mind, I identify in DeBaggio's first narrative the history professor's artistically described 'hypocognitive' state, whereas DeBaggio's second text equals the beginning of the actual performance of this state. This very state then emulates, following Arno Geiger's deliberations, what apparently becomes natural to a 'hypercognitive' society. This is in agreement with Jesse F. Ballenger's observations. Ballenger claims that 'the person with Alzheimer's in social constructionist discourse becomes a veritable prophet of the postmodern self', a notion I take up more fully in Chap. 5. More specifically, Ballenger describes the model of a 'modern self' as viewing a person as a self 'because she knows, in very concrete terms, who, what, and where she is in the world'. A postmodern view of the self, by comparison, considers a person:

> a self when he is connected to a world that will accept him no matter how grave his failings, no matter how confused and forgetful he may be about the particulars of who, what and where he is.[38]

---

[37] DeBaggio's deliberations on death and dying intensify towards the end: following an example of Peter Garrard et al., in 'The effects of very early Alzheimer's disease on the characteristics of writing by a renowned author', *Brain*, 128 (2005), pp. 250–260 (Garrard et al. 2005), a Concordance® word count (http://www.rjcw.freeserve.co.uk; May 2011) of the last ten pages of the text reveals 'death' as the most frequently used noun; 'Alzheimer's research advocate Tom DeBaggio dies', http://www.npr.org/2011/02/22/133971224/Alzheimers-Advocate-Thomas-DeBaggio-Dies (accessed August 2016).

[38] Ballenger, *Self, Senility and Alzheimer's Disease*, pp. 186, 184, 173 (Ballenger 2006).

The artistic fragmentation in postmodern works is suggestive of the disruptive effects of Alzheimer's disease on thought, memory and perception. DeBaggio's work could be seen as a literary rendering of his condition that converts autobiographical truth into authority.[39] At the same time, the caregiver's narrative and presentation of disruption then gains meaning beyond that of textually mirrored truth: it builds on the patient's licence, that is, her or his own choice of presentation.

Supporting this interpretation, Bennett Kravitz's recent collection of essays that focuses on the representation of disorders that 'owe their existence to specific economic and cultural conditions of the western world', considers Alzheimer's disease to be:

> portrayed as a postmodern illness, with important cultural implications, most often because we come to understand that the disease attacks the personality – and destroys it – well before it leaves its toll on the body.[40]

Kravitz highlights that both presence and awareness of Alzheimer's disease in society continue to increase. But he carries this insight further, when stressing the intricate link between cultural implications and literary explorations of accelerated memory loss.

For his analysis, Kravitz chooses – once more – John Bayley's *Iris: A Memoir of Iris Murdoch*, and Jonathan Franzen's 'My Father's Brain'.[41] He dissects Franzen's motivation to write as an attempt to come to terms with the father's dissolution as well as his own mortality, and identifies Iris Murdoch's travails as Bayley's core focus. In this way, Kravitz pinpoints two of the central issues caregivers grapple with in their accounts, and further underlines Arno Geiger's view and presentation of his father's condition. With Kravitz's deliberations in mind, I argue that Henderson's and DeBaggio's presentations have laid – each in their own way – the cornerstone for individualist presentations by dementia patients; in some ways writing against, to put it in the words

---

[39] Irene Rose, 'Autistic autobiography or autistic life narrative?', *Journal of Literary Disability*, 2.1 (2008), pp. 44–54, p. 52 (Rose 2008).

[40] Bennett Kravitz, *Representations of Illness in Literature and Film* (Newcastle upon Tyne: Cambridge Scholars Publishing, 2010), pp. 1, 6, 103–119 (Kravitz 2010).

[41] Jonathan Franzen, 'My Father's Brain' [2001], in *How to Be Alone* (London: Fourth Estate, 2010), pp. 7–38 (Franzen 2010).

of Arthur W. Frank, the 'cultural dislike for [chaos] stories'.[42] I presently show that, building on further patient activism and an even further increasing awareness of the condition, the stage is being prepared for truly nonconformist patient presentation. Such presentation accepts and advances, in both form and contents, dementia as a natural part of aging.

COLLABORATIVE WRITING MEETS SOCIETAL NORMS AND POLITICAL INTENTIONS

DeBaggio's choice to present a narrative whose form purposefully witnesses disruption and decline explicitly commands his displaying pain and despair. In addition, he enters a harshly reifying discourse, against which other patients before him fervently rebel. His presentation certainly builds on their portrayals as well as the societally slowly changing perception of the still productive patient – I am thinking about Davis's continued witnessing, McGowin's social activism and Henderson's participation in a drug trial. The journalist and writer, in turn, contributes with an artful narrative that offers *An Intimate Look at Life with Alzheimer's*. In this understanding, DeBaggio can remain true to himself. He can reveal his vulnerability, and, thus, maintain identity and authority in weakness, even though these characteristics run counter to convictions professed in most illness narratives, namely that, as Kathlyn Conway puts it, 'the right attitude brings a cure'.[43]

In the above discussion, I have variously pointed to the problematic relationship between a triumphalist illness presentation and the chronic degenerative nature of dementia: the cognitive decline in dementia is, not only in medico-scientific terms, perceived of as unidirectional in nature. In this respect, I very much agree with Conway that the societally prescribed adherence to a narrative of triumph can be harmful to the patient, especially, when a walk into the sunrise must remain illusory. If, however, an account achieves the combination – presenting a triumphalist storyline, while offering an exploration of the author-narrator's limits – it may, in formally securing a larger readership, purposefully

---

[42] Frank, *Storyteller*, p. 100 (Frank 1995).
[43] Conway, *Limits of Expression*, p. 6 (Conway 2007).

further necessary sociopolitical discussion. This is what Thomas Graboys's narrative achieves.[44]

The Harvard cardiologist has Parkinson's disease. Even though the condition is, first and foremost, perceived as a movement disorder, it can, as in Graboys's not unusual case, have a strong cognitive component: aggressively progressing Lewy body dementia.[45] Graboys relies on collaboration with the journalist Peter Zheutlin, because his 'memory often fails, and trying to organize [his] thoughts is often impossible' (xx). We could read his, so enabled, highly articulate narrative as efforts to maintain his authority as an accomplished professional, especially as he admits that 'this book is a logical extension of my medical career' (xxi). What is more, Graboys reserves, as Conway has identified in triumphalist illness narratives, 'reflection for the end', calling the reader never to 'underestimate the power of positive thinking' (160).[46] Chapter headings do not allude to difficulties imposed by his illness. Instead, they suggest deliberations on 'My Days' (1), 'Love and Marriage' (42), 'Doctors and Patient' (59), 'My Family' (86) or 'Friends' (131) and, lastly, 'A Life Beyond Illness' (175), that is, the space 'between the limbo of illness and the anger and despair it often spawns, [...] a better place – a life beyond illness still to be lived' (177).

Nevertheless, 'obsessed and fearful about the progression of the disease and always alert for any changes that might signal an advance of the illness' (151), Graboys talks about his fears directly in the second to last chapter, 'End Game' (161). Affected by how 'both [his] parents suffered from dementia' (163), Graboys is particularly concerned about having an illness 'in which physical death is not necessarily the endpoint [... because he] could linger in the shadows of dementia for many years' (165). Consequently, he openly ponders ethical questions such as:

> Who is to say how much dementia is too much to live with? Who will know what really goes on in my head when I lose the ability to communicate? [...] how exactly – both medically and legally – does one go about ending a

---

[44] Thomas Graboys with Peter Zheutlin, *Life in the Balance. A Physician's Memoir of Life, Love, and Loss with Parkinson's Disease and Dementia* (New York: Sterling Publishing, 2008) (Graboys 2008); references incorporated in the text.

[45] See, e.g., Kurt A. Jellinger, 'Neurobiology of cognitive impairment in Parkinson's disease', *Expert Review of Neurotherapeutics*, 12.12 (2012), pp. 1451–1466 (Jellinger 2012).

[46] Conway, *Limits of Expression*, p. 1 (Conway 2007).

life when the body is intact but the mind is gone? [...] How will I know when the time is right? (166–167)

These are issues that, notably, Walter Jens had been discussing at length with the theologian Hans Küng, long before he was diagnosed with dementia.[47] Mindful of these prominently published insights, Jens and his wife had signed an advanced directive in 2006, two years after the scholar's diagnosis. But, as Inge Jens confesses (and Graboys anticipates):

> Ich weiß es so wenig [...] ob es wirklich Todeswünsche sind, wenn er wiederholt und sehr deutlich artikuliert: 'Ich will nicht mehr', 'Ich möchte tot sein', 'Bitte, lass mich sterben'.
>
> [I know so little whether they are really wishes to die, when he repeatedly and very clearly articulates: 'I don't want any more', 'I want to be dead', 'Please let me die'.][48]

These questions are as pressing as they are distressing. In 1990, a patient could, thinking back to Cohen's argument, bring these questions to the reader only through their dying. Two decades later, patients have gathered pace: Graboys can raise this issue from the vantage point of an authority with the condition; as both doctor and patient. In addition, he follows his understanding, which resonates with Conway's own deliberations, that:

> People always want to read stories of triumph over tragedy. But there is no sugarcoating Parkinson's and, as the baby boomers age and live longer, more and more of us are succumbing to the disease. There is no silver lining here. There is anger, pain, and frustration at being victimized by a disease that can, to some extent, be managed but cannot be cured. (xviii)

In our increasing appreciation of the patient's continued self and identity within their condition, we should take particular note of these quandaries, openly deliberate on their ethical tenability – and hear patients out in *all* their concerns and bring them in relation to the caregivers' view.

---

[47] Walter Jens and Hans Küng, *Menschenwürdig sterben. Ein Plädoyer für Selbstverantwortung* [Dying in dignity. An appeal for personal responsibility] [1995] (Munich: Piper, 2009) (Jens and Küng 2009).

[48] Jens, *Unvollständige Erinnerungen*, p. 300 (I. Jens 2009).

Surely, Graboys's closing with 'a search for hope and courage' (178) could, next to being read as the note of a 'survivor', be interpreted as fitting into mainstream conceptualisations of masculinity. The formal layout of this book suggests that I perceive of the caregiver discourse as much more evidently gendered than the patient discourse. Still, we are compelled to ask, whether male as compared to female patients generally portray their condition differently; whether such a difference goes beyond the telling of a purportedly seamless narrative, the artistic exploitation of their condition, or the formal underplaying of their concerns. In Chap. 5, I look at narratives offered by patients who published their stories once the Alzheimer's patient movement had fully taken off. This gives me the opportunity to investigate more deeply whether the patient discourse is as strictly gendered as the caregiver discourse seems to be, and whether there are forms of dementia life-writing that enable patients to remain true to their narrative abilities, bringing poetics and politics in unison.

Open Access This chapter is distributed under the terms of the Creative Commons Attribution 4.0 International License (http://creativecommons.org/licenses/by/4.0/), which permits use, duplication, adaptation, distribution and reproduction in any medium or format, as long as you give appropriate credit to the original author(s) and the source, a link is provided to the Creative Commons license and any changes made are indicated.

The images or other third party material in this chapter are included in the work's Creative Commons license, unless indicated otherwise in the credit line; if such material is not included in the work's Creative Commons license and the respective action is not permitted by statutory regulation, users will need to obtain permission from the license holder to duplicate, adapt or reproduce the material.

CHAPTER 5

On Reclaiming Authority: The Enabling Discourse of Alzheimer's Disease

Abstract This chapter illustrates how more recent Alzheimer's disease patient narratives take patient activism further in both form and contents. Disease-imposed constraints become the narrative's core in terms of both aesthetic presentation and political pursuit. This development parallels the changes observed in caregiver life-writing, as patients and their needs reach the centre of narrative presentation and performance. This chapter argues that patients can thrive, building on earlier advocacy of their fellow sufferers, on more fragmented illness presentation. They can choose narrative forms that match their attention span as well as their political intentions, and show them as living within their remaining capabilities. In this way, patients authoritatively claim their continued independence within their narrative abilities, making themselves partners in the ensuing sociopolitical, cultural and economic debates.

Keywords Diary · Essay · Illness performance · Patient authority · Postmodern identity

© The Author(s) 2017
M. Zimmermann, *The Poetics and Politics of Alzheimer's Disease Life-Writing*, Palgrave Studies in Literature, Science and Medicine, DOI 10.1007/978-3-319-44388-1_5

I was just tired of people labeling me as crazy and not trying to understand the disease or support me.[1]

Alzheimer ist zwar eine harte Sache – aber weil es eben auch so hart ist, habe ich das Gefühl, vor nichts mehr Angst haben zu müssen. Und das eröffnet Möglichkeiten und Chancen.

[Alzheimer's is a tough thing – but since it is so tough, I feel I don't have to be afraid of anything anymore. And this opens up opportunities and chances.][2]

Patrick McDonagh has offered a detailed analysis of the representation of idiocy and folly as genealogical precursors of intellectual or cognitive disability. In drawing on popular, scientific, sociopolitical and literary discourses, his work suggests that not only cultural traditions, as identified by Woodward, but especially also economic considerations and demographic structures impact on how society views mental disability. McDonagh projects his insights into conceptual developments in nineteenth-century Britain onto the present-day representation of 'people identified as having intellectual or learning disabilities'.[3] He places significant emphasis on institutional criticism and socio-economic considerations, thus, inviting a deliberation on the growing prevalence of older age cognitive impairment in modern times.

In the preceding chapter, I highlighted how the perceived societal pressure to perform as an able social being impacts on the author-narrators' choice of presentation, likely at the expense of an account that would be fully credible in narrative terms. At the same time, we have become aware of a slow shift towards accounts that increasingly embrace the disease's impact on narrative capabilities. Two moves have taken place: first, the step from traditionalist linear storylines to accounts that accept disease-imposed narrative fragmentation as a given; and, thereafter, the step towards the patient's deliberate choice of fragmented narration. This second move suggests that a new 'norm' has entered patient life-writing and articulation – a fact I almost see in ironic contradistinction to

---

[1] Mobley, *Young Hope*, p. 13 (Mobley 2007).

[2] Christian Zimmermann and Peter Wißmann, *Auf dem Weg mit Alzheimer. Wie sich mit einer Demenz leben lässt* [On the road with Alzheimer's. How it is possible to live with dementia] (Frankfurt am Main: Mabuse-Verlag, 2011), p. 47 (Zimmermann and Wißmann 2011).

[3] Patrick McDonagh, *Idiocy. A Cultural History* (Liverpool: Liverpool University Press, 2008), p. 336 (McDonagh 2008).

Ramanathan's remark that patients elaborate their telling in negotiation with their audience 'like those of us who are normal'.[4]

Ramanathan made this observation in 1997, two years after Lennard J. Davis had asserted that 'our construction of the normal world is based on a radical repression of disability'. Davis specifically concentrates on the physical body, but his brief excursion on madness as a condition that similarly 'shows up as a disruption in the visual field' makes his work directly applicable to cognitive decline:

> [T]he fear is that the mind is fragmenting, breaking up, falling apart, losing itself – all terms we associate with becoming mad. With the considerable information we have about the biological roots of mental illness, we begin to see the disease again as a breaking up of 'normal' body chemistry: amino acid production gone awry, depleted levels of certain polypeptide chains or hormones.[5]

Henderson's as well as DeBaggio's outspoken and deliberate choice to tell the disease in an unconventional, a not 'normal' form reflects a shift in power structures. This shift increasingly enables patients to tell their story within a new framework of narrative norms; norms that do not demand temporal coherence or romantic endings for an individual self and continued personhood to be acknowledged by a reader who, in refusing such acknowledgement, as Davis would put it, remains an 'outsider'.

In this final chapter, I look at patient narratives that have emerged against the background of, and in mutual exchange with, such shifting power structures. I particularly analyse the reflections of recently rising patient activism in first-person testimonies. With McDonagh's observations in mind, I hope to identify how patients assert themselves in the context of increasing socio-economic and healthcare pressures, and show how the growing societal awareness of the condition influenced patient writing. My comparison of Jeanne L. Lee's and Richard Taylor's accounts deliberates once more on how gender influences the formal means these author-narrators choose to assert their continued identity within such a shifting discourse.

In the second part of this chapter, I read Claude Couturier's diary and Christine Bryden's collage with the question in mind as to how their

---

[4] Ramanathan, *Alzheimer Discourse*, p. 70 (see above p. 77) (Ramanathan 1997).
[5] Lennard J. Davis, *Enforcing Normalcy. Disability, Deafness, and the Body* (London: Verso, 1995), pp. 22, 142 (Davis 1995).

presentations bring together a drive to counter-narrate societal perceptions of passivity and dependence, on the one hand, and an awareness of the necessity to offer a readable account that nevertheless accepts disease-imposed limitations, on the other hand. I argue that the essay or diary entry as narrative forms that match the patient's short attention span, while pre-empting the need for closure, unite poetic possibilities and political necessities for patients to dictate changes in a shifting dementia discourse.

I close this chapter asking how the 'genre' of dementia patient narratives has evolved, and in what ways this development parallels that observed for dementia caregiver narratives. To this end, I reflect on a narrative, whose publication has been championed by a patient support network. This link echoes the political nature of Sylvia Zacharias's publication with and for Hirnliga ten years earlier. Helga Rohra acknowledges her narrative limits, but, as the acknowledged speaker of an organised patient movement, sets the bar high for political and socio-economic change.

Times Are Changing II: Patient Activism

Founding member of DASNI, Jeanne L. Lee freely admits the struggles of bringing her story to paper:

> I looked back on my notes and realized that even I couldn't figure out what was what, so how could I expect anyone else to be able to decipher all those mumbo jumbo notes? [. . .] I began to do more on my tape recorder [. . .]. I just had to do it, because I was afraid that if I didn't get the thought down right then, I would forget [. . .].[6]

As the discrepancy between the eloquent presentation and her professed cognitive difficulties suggests, Lee had to engage the professional writer Cliff Reid to bring her story to print. Reid openly confesses that the notes 'were quite honestly scary. The tapes were [. . .] somewhat disorganized and repetitive' (77), echoing the impressions we gain from

---

[6] Lee, *Just Love Me*, p. 50 (Lee 2003); all further references incorporated in the text; see the DASNI document http://www.dasninternational.org/2011/DASNI_A5_12pp_Final.pdf (accessed August 2016), with short biographies of founding members.

Henderson's repetitive journal entries. All the same, going to this enormous trouble supports the notion that such writing is to be taken seriously in its exceptionality, especially since the few voices that come to articulate their concerns are the ones advocating for the community of their fellow sufferers, who remain silent.[7] As I emphasised previously, I believe that patient accounts deserve particular attention, given the tension between current health and social care policies, on the one hand, and the core issues that these patients are crucially concerned with, on the other hand: the medication of their cognitive decline, a working doctor–patient relationship or, as in Graboys's case, end-of-life questions.[8]

On an aesthetic level, however, collaborative composition makes it difficult to rely on stylistic choices for getting to grips with Lee's perception of her condition. Therefore, I prefer to focus on the contents of her narrative, also because she claims to:

> have personally reviewed every word that appears on these pages [...] to ensure that this book represents a credible journey through the emotional world of someone actually afflicted with the disease. (xviii)

What is more, to add further credibility to her telling, Lee supplements, similar to Graboys, her narrative with letters from family and friends. While their selection remains Lee's prerogative, family loyalty should be assumed as a given.

Lee's journey formulation relies on her learning to come to terms with her diagnosis. She openly admits her memory lapses, failed marriages, alcohol and drug abuse, and 'one long succession of suicide attempts' (20). Eventually, she considers the 'Alzheimer's diagnosis to be the best news I'd heard in my life' (23), since she now 'could quit trying so hard to cover up my forgetfulness' (23). I see Lee's embracing her diagnosis as the final rescue from a life that lacked focus. In this spirit, over two thirds of her text are dedicated to bringing out her activist nature and her

---

[7] Patricia Haas Stanley, 'The patient's voice: a cry in solitude or a call for community', *Literature and Medicine*, 23.2 (2004), pp. 346–363 (Stanley 2004).

[8] Martina Zimmermann, 'Dementia in life-writing: our health care system in the words of the sufferer', *Neurological Sciences*, 32 (2011), pp. 1233–1238 (Zimmermann 2011).

acceptance of the condition. Both are strongly reflected in her desire 'to help improve the understanding between people with Alzheimer's and those who interact with them' (xviii), and are lived out in her dedicating entire chapters to 'doing what I can' (37), or 'doctors and health' (53).

While such emphasis on significance may be rooted in Reid's efforts to structure Lee's notes, it further underlines Lee's agency. This agency counter-narrates Jean Grothé's passive presentation of his mother which is governed by the concept of decline. Lee follows the insight that: 'The past is just our experience, and hopefully what we have learned from our experience will lead us to live this moment, right now, in a better way' (71). This appreciation echoes Christian Zimmermann's above-quoted view of his condition or Arno Geiger's perception of his father's continued, experience-shaped personality. It comes from the understanding 'that the future, near the end of life, will ultimately take care of itself and is not worth worrying about'.[9] Lee's journey leads her, as Ryan and colleagues would say, to 'a new kind of spiritual awareness'.[10]

According to Robert Hill, this present-focused adapting supports coping with cognitive decline much more effectively than concentrating on the past as such – as seen in the accounts of female adult-child caregivers. Such observations further enhance our understanding, gained from an analysis of Phillip Toledano's and Arno Geiger's presentations, that the positive conceptualisation of Alzheimer's disease is intricately linked to that of aging itself. I shall return to this question further below, exploring as to how patients may assert themselves against preconceptions of Alzheimer's disease as a condition of old age.

In comparison to Robert Davis, Diana Friel McGowin or Larry Rose, Jeanne L. Lee admits to her condition very openly, embraces her diagnosis with optimism and readily surrenders to the need for help in writing her narrative. This attitude may at least partly rely on the fact that dementia has become much more present in the public domain and that caregiving approaches increasingly focus on the wellbeing and continued identity of the patient. Still, I keep wondering, mindful of Graboy's or DeBaggio's presentations, whether Lee's choice of presentation is also related to her writing as a female patient. Turning to a male activist-patient's account will hopefully give some answers.

---

[9] Hill, *Positive Aging*, p. 28 (Hill 2005).
[10] Ryan, Bannister and Anas, 'The dementia narrative', p. 150 (Ryan et al. 2009).

In stark contrast to several of the narratives discussed so far, Richard Taylor's text is not a print-on-demand, let alone self-funded publication, but marketed by a medical publisher.[11] Taylor is promoted as an authority, who addresses, as the cover promises, 'the complexity and emotions surrounding issues such as the loss of independence and personhood, unwanted personality shifts, the struggle to communicate', '[w]ith poignant clarity, candor, and humor'. In short, Taylor speaks 'from the inside' in a large-size volume that rather aspires to a degree-course textbook than an engaging paperback.

In purposeful unison with the objective of this presentation, the systematic classification of Taylor's essays precludes the depiction of his gradual decline, while their brevity meets the limitation of short attention span. Likewise, a collection of essays skilfully circumvents the lack of happy closure; it does not follow the traditional narrative convention to 'restructure past memories and future expectations in a way that would cohere with the present, bridging the gap by creating a new kind of continuity'.[12]

Also in using a highly accomplished tone that hardly gives cognitive challenge away (but likely suggests editorial support), Taylor claims the intellectual agility that Tilman Jens denies his father. In addition, he frequently describes his condition in terms of a jokey personification, illustrating 'Dr. Alzheimer and his gang of sticky-footed ne'er-do-wells [as] tromp[ing] around my brain' (xvi) or on an 'extended visit between my ears' (xviii). Such self-deprecating, sarcastic irony suggests that he experiences his condition beyond feelings of anger and resentment. He plays down the actually occurring loss of nerve cells by using euphemisms that conjecture local and, hence, emotional distance from the intellect-threatening centre of the illness process.

That said, Taylor's book provides a powerful platform for his engagement in a patient-centred discourse. Of course, he only can enter the debate in this authoritative form against the background of twenty-five years of lived, gradually intensified and socially accepted Alzheimer's patient activism. Until his death in July 2015, Taylor was an active

---

[11] Richard Taylor, *Alzheimer's from the Inside Out* (Baltimore: Health Professions Press, 2007) (Taylor 2007); references incorporated in the text.
[12] Shlomith Rimmon-Kenan, 'The story of "I": illness and narrative identity', *Narrative*, 10.1 (2002), pp. 9–27, p. 13 (Rimmon-Kenan 2002).

member of DASNI and ADI.[13] Their establishing is rooted in the writing of patients like McGowin and Rose who called for patient representation and support, and the active contributions of patients like Lee. At the same time, Taylor writes in the awareness and confidence of increasingly promoted patient-centred care. This observation is in line with Basting's deliberations on Richard Taylor, whom she considers a representative of the 'new generation of dementia activists' who build on the foundations of earlier patients. It is of particular note then that Basting, who had personal e-mail exchange with Taylor, considered his book, compared to his e-mails, 'rather tame'.[14]

Amongst others, the psychologist carves out the linguistic subtleties pertaining to a politically correct Alzheimer's discourse, and aims to re-establish his subjectivity in the face of infantilising and reifying treatment. For example, he stresses that '[t]he fact that I have a disease affecting my memory and cognitive processes does not make me any less an adult or any more like a child' (189), coming to literally shout at the reader: 'I am not a child. Even if sometimes I act like one, check me out – I AM NOT A CHILD!' (190; emphasis original). But still, Taylor indirectly links, reminiscent of Reeve Lindbergh's illustrations, his own behaviour to that of a child, when, for example, juxtaposing his granddaughter's 'early childhood reality' to his own being 'confused by fantasy [...] and reality' (154).

In partially surrendering to such disabling discourse, Taylor signals his speechlessness in the confrontation with an elusive disease process. Equally, the very tension between private experience and public expression plainly epitomises the fear of losing his standing as a mind-defined psychologist, and echoes the formal and contextual conflicts perceived in Thomas Graboys's memoir. It also dismantles Taylor's self-affirming strategy as only partly suitable in view of the condition's progressive nature. In line with this observation and based on the insight that especially male illness stories must offer the narrator 'some compensatory power and freedom', I believe the positive, less intellect-focused presentation in the earlier male narratives to be rooted in the fact that

---

[13] Alzheimer's Disease International, 'In memory of Richard Taylor', http://www.alz.co.uk/news/in-memory-of-richard-taylor-phd (accessed August 2016).
[14] Basting, *Forget Memory*, pp. 145–153, esp. pp. 152, 149 (Basting 2009).

their narrators interpret themselves as justifiably guided or impaired for a higher purpose.[15] In making this claim, I am very much aware that the sample is, though unavoidably, small; but Robert Davis's, Charles Schneider's and Larry Rose's positive outlook is faith-related, as is Mike Donohue's view professed in his pathography.[16]

As Taylor struggles to reconcile his narrative choices fully with the chronic degenerative nature of his condition, we continue to wonder how patients may assert themselves in a discourse that strongly relies on conceptualisations of Alzheimer's disease as a condition of old age. This question becomes particularly pressing in the light of Robert Hill's above-discussed insights that lead me to think that the positive conceptualisation of Alzheimer's disease is tied to that of aging itself.

Two further texts carry such an enabling notion of Alzheimer's patient discourse a long way: they are written by activist-patients, who strongly identify themselves in their condition, both in terms of the attitudes they profess and the narrative forms they choose. These texts challenge the societal perception of females as being passive and dependent – especially in the confrontation with a condition that is perceived as compromising the male-associated mind more than the female-associated body.

Identity within Dementia: The Patient as Postmodern Prophet?

The title of Christine Bryden's book, *Dancing with Dementia*, anticipates that her narrative does not fit the concept of quest or chaos narrative.[17] Indeed, the story begins with Bryden (formerly Boden) taking up studies and getting remarried in the light of her Alzheimer's disease diagnosis having been amended to that of less aggressively

---

[15] Couser, *Recovering Bodies*, p. 185 (Couser 1997).
[16] Mike Donohue, *From AA to AD, a Wistful Travelogue* (Seattle: CreateSpace, 2009) (Donohue 2009); see also: Jon C. Stuckey, 'Blessed assurance. The role of religion and spirituality in Alzheimer's disease caregiving and other significant life events', *Journal of Aging Studies*, 15 (2001), pp. 69–84 (Stuckey 2001).
[17] Christine Bryden, *Dancing with Dementia. My Story of Living Positively with Dementia* (London: Jessica Kingsley Publishers, 2005) (Bryden 2005); references incorporated in the text.

advancing frontotemporal dementia.[18] Therefore, one is tempted to read her narrative as the story of her rebirth. In the first place, this rebirth is not related to her strengthened faith: as a practising Christian, Bryden refrains, in agreement with Hawkins's findings, from using religious metaphors or myths. Rather, Bryden's sense of renewal is closely linked to the perception of having survived the life-threatening diagnosis of Alzheimer's disease, whose confrontation she had described in her first book that largely follows the traditional journey myth.[19]

These first impressions of Bryden's narrative are in tune with Jessica Kingsley's assertion that 'she only ever prints an autobiographical narrative that has something different to say, something that cannot be found elsewhere'.[20] In fact, Bryden's metaphorical conceptualisation of 'rising like a phoenix out of the ashes of that terrible time' (164) adds a further, unexpected perspective to our reading of the narratives explored so far. It highlights the threat that patients like Robert Davis or Thomas DeBaggio feel. This very different notion is particularly tangible, because Bryden's initial view of the diagnosis as tantamount to a '[d]eath by small steps' changes to that of an 'identity crisis' (156) – a move that alters her quality of life notably.[21]

Against this background, Bryden's metaphorical language belongs to a journey from which she could *actually* return; and her shifted outlook gives new meaning to what we have come to understand as disabling images. She requests her fellow sufferers as well as caregivers to:

> find the pearl hidden within us. Like the pearl that is formed through the irritation of a grain of sand within an oyster, our pearl has formed through the challenge of living with dementia. (168)

This invitation gives the shell the entirely different notion of value and growth. Patients like Thomas DeBaggio, or caregivers like Frank Wall, by

---

[18] Nancy A. Pachana et al., 'Comparison of neuropsychological functioning in Alzheimer's disease and frontotemporal dementia', *Journal of the International Neuropsychological Society*, 2 (1996), pp. 505–510 (Pachana et al. 1996).

[19] Boden, *Who Will I Be When I Die?* (Boden 1998).

[20] Rose, 'Autistic autobiography', p. 52 (Rose 2008).

[21] Boden, *Who Will I Be When I Die?*, p. 48 (Boden 1998); Couser made a similar observation in relation to HIV/AIDS narratives; see: *Recovering Bodies*, pp. 82–84 (Couser 1997).

comparison, see this shell as empty and, thus, use it as an image of the patient's lost potential. Undoubtedly, Robert Davis and others describe a learning process, but their accounts lack Bryden's metaphorical emphasis on surprise, which further accentuates their desperation. The same is true for Bryden's affirmation that '[e]ach person with dementia is as worthy and precious as a beautiful newborn baby, a gift for us all to cherish' (170). This view counters Spohr's objectifying or Ernaux's helpless use of the child metaphor; and it brings out how differently Bryden perceives of her situation as compared to Taylor. But it also illustrates how strongly metaphorical language relies on the context in which it develops.[22]

Bryden's inferred emphasis on the patient as being the opportunity of growth and development reaches far beyond the perception of McGowin's, Lee's or, indeed, Taylor's 'still being able' as counteracting the disabling notions of the child metaphor. Her conceptualisation of growth is necessarily linked to her retrospectively working through the illness experience, with the second chance giving her the opportunity to live out her gratitude. Such a reading adds to a positive reception of her narrative, as gratitude is considered an optimistic coping strategy in the confrontation with age-related decline.[23]

But Bryden's linguistically suggested presence is only partially reflected in the dynamics of her narrative that sets out to chronicle her frequent journeys to support DASNI and ADI, but then mutates into a collection of revised talks she had given during these trips. These essays relate '[w]hat it feels like to live with dementia' (97) or the 'many ways to help' (122), and, thus, excellently lend themselves to teaching good pharmaceutical care. Together with further information-containing appendices, these essays encompass over half of the book. Alluding to Taylor's formal choices, this arrangement confirms Bryden's ongoing cognitive challenges, to which she, however, owns up very openly:

> It has been a tremendous struggle to collect together all my thoughts, talks, speeches, correspondence, notes and so on, for the last six years. Inspiration, rather than memory, has been the thread that enabled me to weave these disjointed fragments into this book. (173)

[22] Simi Linton, 'Reassigning meaning', in *The Disability Studies Reader*, ed. by Davis, pp. 223–236 (Linton 2010).
[23] Hill, *Positive Aging*, pp. 169–175 (Hill 2005).

As such, the book's composition demonstrates, yet again, that '"self" is more than memory'.[24] This is especially true since we identify what Anthony Elliot would describe as Bryden's 'floating in a realm of fleeting moments, transitory encounters, eternal presents' as a harmonious adapting to her memory loss.[25] Indeed, Bryden's narrative articulates, in both form and contents, what Elliot defines, and Ballenger deliberates on, as 'postmodern self'. The very combination of reflective essay with agency inspiring travel reports embodies the continuing surprises in Alzheimer's patients, without slipping into a romanticising survivor mentality. Bryden concludes:

> It is time to move away from the bright lights to a corner of the floor where the rhythm is slower and the music quieter, but still sweet. All I can do now is sit quietly and listen, and hope for a cure. (174)

In the context of Bryden's dance metaphor I think it noteworthy that Kingsley Publishers cover Bryden's text with abstract, dance inspiring motifs in bright colours that match the shirt Bryden wears on the inset photo. While other book jackets display faded photographs (McGowin) or half the face of their author-narrator (DeBaggio, Henderson) or designs alluding to the journey into the sunset or a variation thereof (Rose, Davis, Donohue), this design very much suggests Bryden's active involvement in this dance and underlines her life-affirming attitude.[26]

Yet, in view of Bryden's sustained activities, the argument could now run that she finds these powerful images – and carries DeBaggio's postmodern description on a lived level – principally based on her altered diagnosis and the cognitive changes related to her type of dementia.[27] Patients suffering from frontotemporal dementia can, indeed, undergo

---

[24] Boyd H. Davis, 'Introduction: some commonalities', in *Alzheimer Talk, Text and Context. Enhancing Communication*, ed. by Boyd H. Davis (New York: Palgrave Macmillan, 2008), pp. xi–xxi, p. xvi (Davis 2008); and therein: Dena Shenk, 'There was an old woman: maintenance of identity by people with Alzheimer's dementia', pp. 3–17 (Shenk 2008).

[25] Anthony Elliott, *Concepts of the Self* (Cambridge: Polity Press, 2008), p. 154 (Elliott 2008).

[26] See also: Annette Leibing, 'Divided gazes. Alzheimer's disease, the person within, and death in life', in *Thinking about Dementia*, ed. by Leibing and Cohen, pp. 240–268, pp. 253, 259, 263 fn. 19 (Leibing 2006); and Jane Wilkinson, 'Remembering forgetting', *Status Quaestionis*, 6 (2014), pp. 103–121, p. 107 (Wilkinson 2014).

[27] See also her internet presence: 'Christine Bryden. Dementia from an insider's perspective', http://www.christinebryden.com/ (accessed August 2016).

profound personality changes, and this may be reflected in their developing specific artistic talent.[28] But such cases are equally seen in Alzheimer's disease, where art therapy supports the patient's wellbeing and communication.[29] Claude Couturier's diary affirms such considerations.[30]

At the core of her narrative fragments lies a dry humour – possibly reminiscent of Spohr's certain detachment – that challenges, in Bryden's spirit, the traditional use of metaphors. Couturier is, for example, concerned about ending up in a vegetative state, an 'existence... de légume' [vegetable existence], and would much rather 'être incinérée' [be incinerated] under such circumstances.[31] Nevertheless, she continues with 'je serai un légume grillé' [I will be a grilled vegetable; 71], which pokes fun at such inanimate discourse. What is more, in hoping that 'Dieu au moins sait ce que deviennent mes neurones disparus, et surtout qu'il en fait un bon usage' [God at least knows what becomes of my lost neurons and that, above all, he makes good use of them; 72], she lifts the cause of her memory loss onto a literally unreachable level. This strategy implies her unspoken acceptance that there is – in view of the illness's terminal nature – no battle to be fought. The self-saving power of this image starkly contrasts the living death or death sentence, which precludes the option of battle for Thomas DeBaggio, Walter Jens and others and, additionally, deprives them of any activity outside such battle.

Couturier's continued agency is revealed in her artistic creativity, demonstrated in eight of her paintings that are reproduced on glossy paper in the centre of her diary. Works dating from early stages of her condition, such as 'Soleils de nuit' [Sunflowers at night] reflect, as do their titles, Couturier's painful awareness of her condition. She expresses this awareness as 'des instants de lucidité terribles, où l'immensité de mon angoisse prend le dessus quand je vois l'étendue de la dégradation de mes facultés dites

---

[28] See, for example, Tiffany W. Chow, 'Personality in frontal lobe disorders', *Current Psychiatry Reports*, 2.5 (2000), pp. 446–451 (Chow 2000); Bruce L. Miller et al., 'Emergence of artistic talent in frontotemporal dementia', *Neurology*, 51 (1998), pp. 978–981 (Miller et al. 1998).

[29] See, for example, Carlos H. Espinel, 'de Kooning's late colours and forms: dementia, creativity, and the healing power of art', *The Lancet*, 347 (1996), pp. 1096–1098 (Espinel 1996).

[30] Claude Couturier, *Puzzle. Journal d'une Alzheimer* [Jigsaw. Diary of an Alzheimer's patient] (Paris: Josette Lyon, 2004) (Couturier 2004); references incorporated in the text.

[31] 'Incinéré' can be translated as 'incinerated' or 'cremated', the latter refering to subjects, the former rather to objects; for Couturier's use of metaphors, see: Zimmermann, 'Alzheimer's disease metaphors' (Zimmermann forthcoming).

"normales"' [moments of terrible clarity, when the immensity of my anxiety is overwhelming, as I see the extent of the degeneration of my so-called 'normal' abilities; 103]. The painting's few colours and sharp contours mark the harsh contrast between Couturier's 'sunlit' awareness within the illness-associated darkness. But as Couturier incorporates Robert Davis's image into her own creativity and continued autonomy, she works through the frightening outlook proposed by the metaphor itself.[32]

All the same, her deliberations emphasise that her journal provides the means for coping on a daily basis. Her diary may be seen as the true literary counterpart of the degenerative nature of the illness, not least since both narrator and reader live with the condition's uncertainty within the narrator's horizon and narrative abilities.[33] This is especially true, when considering that, in comparison, Henderson's diary-like fragments are framed by his wife's retrospective deliberations on his state. One could caution that Couturier may have revised or significantly altered her diary before handing it to the publisher so that its credibility in reflecting day-to-day changes may be undermined. However, she was prompted on potential publication by her doctor only eight years into her writing, when substantial revision would have been difficult in view of her more advanced cognitive challenge.[34] Most importantly, the comparison to Henderson's memoir illuminates how drastically publishers' understanding of the readership's acceptance of postmodern narrative forms has advanced. It also highlights, again, the changing perception patients themselves have of their situation and position of authority within society.

I see this observation supported when revisiting my discussion of Annie Ernaux's notes. The diary explicitly includes the prospect of death, instead of searching for false closure, like, for example, Thomas DeBaggio's illness-mirroring text. In line with these considerations, Couturier's later

---

[32] Ruth Abraham offers suggestions for interpretation of patient art work, in *When Words Have Lost Their Meaning. Alzheimer's Patients Communicate through Art* (Westport: Praeger, 2005), esp. pp. 68–81, 105–138 (Abraham 2005).

[33] Consider also Couser's observations on the congruence between the reader's expectation of a terminally ill patient and the form of diary that admits death as a possibility and prospect; see: *Recovering Bodies*, p. 65 (Couser 1997).

[34] Pascale Krémer, 'Alzheimer. Récits d'un exil intérieur', *Le Monde 2*, 20 October 2007 (Krémer 2007); see also Couturier's forum: http://fr.groups.yahoo.com/group/vivremalgre_alzheimer/, which was initiated in May 2004; it continued to be active when I accessed it in August 2013, but was inactive by November 2015.

paintings can be read as a window onto her increasing preoccupations and changing mind set. 'Sortir' [Leaving] is composed of pastel, though still bright colours, and artistically witnesses Couturier's decline, because its impressionistic style focuses less on detail. Likewise, her motif anticipates the advanced condition, given that '[l]andscapes present a simple and satisfying theme'. In fact, since this painting depicts a stony road winding past a protruding panorama of trees in bloom, towards towering mountains, the onlooker perceives of Couturier as picturing her experience in a manner, reminiscent of McGowin's presentation, as a journey towards the unknown, fully aware of her daily struggles and ambivalence.[35]

It is noteworthy in this context that the daughter Kim Howes Zabbia portrays her mother's condition in expressionistic terms, relying on mute and deep colours.[36] This choice may well suggest her inability to understand the mother's state. Couturier, by comparison, demonstrates continued realistic agency mostly relying on impressionistic style. This discrepancy, again, highlights the difference in viewpoint and perception between caregiver and patient.

Ultimately, Couturier and Bryden demonstrate that Alzheimer's disease affects each individual in different ways, even releasing originality and creativity. They both embody the deeper meaning of Toledano's 'river', as they live out their identity beyond the diagnosis, unconcerned about the distance to its 'mouth'. Admittedly, both patients witness to their strong faith, but – in comparison to the believers Rose, Schneider and Davis – they do not devise eventually only partly enabling explanatory strategies in the first place. Instead, they almost come to see their condition and its consequences as integral parts of their lives.

Audacious as it may sound: in the same way as the Alzheimer's condition imposes emotionality, passivity and dependence on its 'victims', these characteristics are moved beyond their traditional classification as only female. The female Alzheimer's story becomes the synthesis of gender- and illness-related conceptualisation. And the female individual with Alzheimer's disease, who demonstrates activity and independence, surmounts both the gender- and illness-related prejudice, to be perceived as doubly strong – exactly like the female caregiver who rises

---

[35] Abraham, *When Words Have Lost Their Meaning*, pp. 71, 112 (Abraham 2005).
[36] Kim Howes Zabbia, *Painted Diaries. A Mother and Daughter's Experience through Alzheimer's* (Minneapolis: Fairview Press, 1996) (Zabbia 1996).

above these ideological prejudices. Framed by the rapidly increasing prevalence and general awareness of the condition, the patient's original need to secure societal respect through assertion of the self in a polished narrative moves towards the awareness of a separate 'Alzheimer's patient identity', who performs and fully lives within the condition and its presentation.[37]

The Patient's World Advises Caregiver and Society

I close my deliberations on narratives by individuals with dementia by looking at a recent publication that, to my mind, not only encompasses the observed changes in the patient discourse but carries the patient self-concept beyond the levels of autonomy discussed so far. The freelance simultaneous translator in the area of medicine and natural sciences Helga Rohra was fifty-five when she was diagnosed with Lewy body dementia.[38] She was the first patient to be elected onto the board of the Munich Alzheimer's Society, which attracted attention from one of Germany's prominent broadsheet newspapers.[39] And her narrative gains particular authority, as its publication was championed by Demenz Support Stuttgart (DSS), whose work furthers 'das Wohlbefinden von Menschen mit Demenz und das ihrer Begleiter' [the wellbeing of individuals with dementia as well as that of their companions].[40] That DSS calls family members companions rather than caregivers inverts the concept underlying earlier approaches of patient-centred care, let alone caregiver-centred attitudes. Patients are considered as continuously independent individuals with a condition.[41]

---

[37] This idea is in line with John Perry's concept of personhood in Alzheimer's disease, as he asserts that 'identities change, in the psychological sense, but they are the same person'; see: 'Diminished and fractured selves', in *Personal Identity and Fractured Selves*, ed. by Mathews, Bok and Rabins, pp. 129–162, p. 149 (Perry 2009).

[38] Helga Rohra, *Aus dem Schatten treten. Warum ich mich für unsere Rechte als Demenzbetroffene einsetze* [Stepping out of the shadow. Why I am advocating our rights as those afflicted by dementia] (Frankfurt am Main: Mabuse-Verlag, 2011) (Rohra 2011); references incorporated in the text.

[39] 'Ich bin dement, na und?' [I am demented, so what?], *Süddeutsche Zeitung*, 1 April 2010.

[40] 'Demenz Support Stuttgart. Philosophie', http://www.demenz-support.de/portraet/philosophie (accessed August 2016).

[41] Basting, *Forget Memory*, presents a powerful collection of examples that 'stress the extent to which [dementia caregiving] is a reciprocal partnership', p. 69 (Basting 2009).

The photograph on the book's front cover embodies this forward-looking illness discourse: Rohra is slightly inclined towards the reader. Peering over her reading glasses, she looks the viewer straight in the eye. Wearing a grey jacket over a dark polo-neck, a pearl necklace as the only accessory, she looks professional, aware, perceptive. We could take this photograph as staged, since Rohra explicitly acknowledges the star photographer Sammy Hart (120). But we come to appreciate it as Rohra's own choice and initiative, when looking at it in the context of her commenting on the approach of a photographer-journalist. After an interview, he requested Rohra to 'sit in front of the window. There I will take some photos of you'. However, Rohra did not like this arrangement. She writes – significantly underpinning earlier considerations regarding Jean Grothé's as compared to Phillip Toledano's presentation of their respective parent:

> Mir gefiel diese Idee jedoch nicht. Bilder von sitzenden, passiven Betroffenen kennen die Leute doch zuhauf. 'Nein, ich will etwas Dynamisches, etwas mit Power. Das Foto soll den Menschen Mut machen.'
>
> [I did not like this idea. People know images of sitting, passive afflicted individuals in droves. 'No, I want something dynamic, something with power. The photo shall inspire people with courage'; 85].

That said, I 'saw' Rohra's subtle and slightly poised smile on the front cover photograph only at a second glance, maybe even only after I had finished reading through her narrative. I wondered whether it was I, the reader and onlooker, who needed time to accept that a dementia patient could still smile, or whether it was Rohra herself who was not totally certain of her emotions. In this context, the double meaning of the title of her narrative is illuminating. 'Stepping out of the shadow' indicates Rohra's reclaiming her right to speak for herself and advocate for her fellow patients – against the common perception that caregivers are the 'only' ones who talk and are heard. This is especially true for the German context, where a dementia patient's popular press first-person account is a first in 2011.[42] This interpretation of Rohra's title, in turn, gains further meaning in the context of Henderson's wish:

---

[42] Next to Rohra's narrative, DSS endorsed Zimmermann and Wißmann, *Auf dem Weg mit Alzheimer* (Zimmermann and Wißmann 2011).

I would love to see some people with Alzheimer's not trying to stay in the shadows all the time but to say, damn it, we're people too. And we want to be talked to and respected as if we were honest to God real people. (7)

Next to depicting the place assigned to patients in the mainstream dementia discourse, Rohra's metaphorical shadow also refers to the illness-related darkness pictured by patients like McGowin or Couturier. Rohra sees herself still stepping outside the condition's metaphorically enhanced liminality. In fact, given that she perceives herself as 'falling' and 'on a slide that leads, in a black tunnel, steep downhill' (37), her 'stepping out of the shadow' is not so dissimilar from Bryden's phoenix image. In this sense, the narrative's title points to a more personal meaning. On an earlier occasion, Rohra had written a book chapter on her illness experience using a pseudonym, because she had not wanted her friends and son to find out about her diagnosis.[43] Owning up to her real name for the purpose of filming at a conference, 'stepping out of the shadow into the limelight' (69) pictures her accepting her life with dementia.[44]

Rohra's portrayal appears so professional that she was suspected not to be a sufferer (92). Mindful of this belittling experience, Rohra is very much aware that her credibility is at stake. She offers reproductions of her handwritten notes that document her earliest shortcomings (19, 27) – echoing Couturier's moment-in-time records. But most of all, Rohra goes to great length to explain her narrative capabilities. Since she seems to anticipate questions of many readers, and responds to what medically focused critics had raised in the context of DeBaggio's narrative, I here quote her at length:

> So leicht es mir fällt, zu erzählen und über meine Erlebnisse zu sprechen, so schwer fällt mir das Schreiben von langen Texten [...]. Wie also sollte aus meinem gesprochenen Wort und meinen kurzen Notizen der Text werden, den Sie heute als Buch in den Händen halten? Die einfachste Lösung wäre

---

[43] Helen Merlin, 'Ich will integriert werden!' [I want to be integrated!], in *'Ich spreche für mich selbst.' Menschen mit Demenz melden sich zu Wort* ['I speak for myself.' People with dementia have their say], ed. by Demenz Support Stuttgart (Frankfurt am Main: Mabuse-Verlag, 2010), pp. 11–24 (Merlin 2010).

[44] A further aspect of growth comes from the fact that Rohra's initial fear that her condition might disrupt the structured, organised and calm environment and rhythm her son, who has Asperger's syndrome, requires, is not confirmed: she comes to realise that her son matures in the confrontation with Rohra's dementia, and their bond becomes even stronger.

ein Ghostwriter gewesen, der wie bei so mancher Autobiografie das Schreiben übernimmt, als Person aber im Verborgenen bleibt. Ein solches Vorgehen kam jedoch weder für mich noch für den Herausgeber oder den Verlag in Frage. Es sollte erst gar nicht der Eindruck entstehen, ich hätte das Buch von Anfang bis Ende allein geschrieben.

[Even if narrating and talking about my experiences comes easily to me, I find it difficult to write long texts (...). But how should my spoken word and short notes become the text, which you now hold as a book in your hands? The simplest solution would have been a ghost writer, who takes on the writing as with so many autobiographies, while remaining hidden in the background. Such a procedure was, however, not acceptable, neither for me nor for the editor nor for the publisher. From the outset we wanted to avoid the impression that I had written the book alone from beginning to end; 11].

Like Jeanne L. Lee's account, Helga Rohra's grew 'nicht am Stück und auch nicht fortlaufend chronologisch, sondern kapitelweise' [not in one piece and also not continuously chronological, but in chapters; 12], with the help of 'Schreibassistenz' [writing assistance]. But in its expository organisation, her narrative still moves from 'the earliest symptoms' (13), 'the first doctor's appointment' (23), to 'the diagnosis' (37), and her 'fight against bureaucracy' (53). Like Tracy Mobley, whom I quote at the beginning of this chapter, she spells out her frustrations with the bureaucratic and social challenges an early-onset patient is confronted with, namely, her battle 'nicht nur gegen die Symptome dieser ungewöhnlichen Demenz, sondern auch gegen die Mühlen der Bürokratie, letztlich ein Kampf ums schlichte Überleben' [not only against the symptoms of this unusual dementia, but also against the grind of bureaucracy, in the end a battle simply for survival; 52]. The condition forces this single mother to give up work, and live on her savings before becoming eligible for social support, and at risk of losing her rented flat. Rohra also finds it difficult to identify a suitable self-help group, because most of them are for caregivers, and the few patient-directed ones are, in view of the condition's demographics, attended by mostly elderly patients. Most of all, however, Rohra laments that:

In Deutschland [gibt es] noch keine Prominenten, die sich zu ihrer Demenz bekennen und als Botschafter für uns sprechen. Wir bräuchten in Deutschland viel mehr Betroffene, die sich als solche zu erkennen geben. Nur so kann sich das allgemeine Bild von Demenz wandeln.

[In Germany, there are no prominent people, who out themselves as suffering from dementia and, thus, speak for us as our ambassadors. We would need many more individuals with the condition in Germany to show themselves as such. Only in this way can the general image of dementia change; 76].

Rudi Assauer's narrative appeared one year later.[45] What could represent the first autobiographical account by a public figure with dementia in Germany, however, reveals itself as a third-person biography of the manager of the Bundesliga football clubs Werder Bremen and Schalke 04. Building on 'zahlreiche persönliche Gespräche mit Rudi Assauer' [numerous personal conversations with Rudi Assauer; 11], the journalist-editor Patrick Strasser eventually decides that:

> Der Gesundheitszustand von Rudi Assauer hat sich über die letzten Monate hinweg verschlechtert, aus diesem Grund habe ich mich gegen einen durchgehenden Erzählstil in der 'Ich-Form' entschieden, da mir eine authentische, detailgetreue Wiedergabe seines Lebens aufgrund seiner Erkrankung an Alzheimer nicht glaubwürdig erschien.
>
> [Rudi Assauer's state of health deteriorated throughout the last few months, therefore, I decided against a consistent narrative style in the 'I-form', as an authentic account, faithful to the detail of his life did not seem believable in view of his Alzheimer's disease; 11].

As Strasser had previously brought out a biography of FC Bayern Munich's (at the time) president, Uli Hoeneß, with the same sport- and lifestyle-oriented publisher, it is not surprising that Assauer's account ends up as a further footballer's biography. The text is, evoking similarity to an interview situation, interspersed by italicised sections that quote Assauer directly. Reminiscent of Taylor's strategy, these sections highlight Assauer's attempts to deflect the serious cognitive implications of his condition, as he mostly refers to his 'Birne' [bulb] rather than brain.[46] All the same, the narrative centrally focuses on the footballer's career, as

---

[45] Rudi Assauer, *Wie ausgewechselt. Verblassende Erinnerungen an mein Leben* [Like substituted. Fading memories of my life] (Munich: Riva, 2012) (Assauer 2012); references incorporated in the text; 'ausgewechselt' can refer to a substitution, for example, in football, but it also has the meaning of 'being changed'.

[46] 'Bulb' refers to the literal translation of 'Birne', which is of colloquial use.

only the first and last chapters explore more fully 'My life with the illness' (17), and 'My women, my future' (229).

However, the footballer started the initiative 'Demenz und Gesellschaft' [Dementia and society], which aims at popularising the condition.[47] Also Rohra continues to be a prominent activist-patient, with media attention to her story and continued activity, 'as if she had made her dementia her profession' (106).[48] Tilman Jens's two narratives certainly provoked heated discussions, but these debates unavoidably centred on the ethics of patient presentation as such. Rohra's text, by comparison, directs attention to the patient's world as well as the need of self-help support to extend continued activity in midlife for as long as possible, while Assauer's public profile aided his cause.

In this context, it cannot be acknowledged and overemphasised enough that the caregiver is most of the time nursing a patient suffering from late-onset dementia in an elderly patient. In addition, the adult child's or spouse's portrayal inevitably reflects the relative's progressed cognitive impairment and concomitant need for guardianship. This, in turn, is – as to be expected – embedded in the caregivers' presentation of their own perceived physical and emotional burden. Early-onset dementia and milder cognitive impairment, in contrast, are usually presented by patients in their midlife themselves.

This comparison of accounts relating to (patient-told) early-stage versus (carer-told) late-stage dementia has highlighted that the former point to the patient's independence, understanding and drive to write and act. Such insights contribute to a less despondent view of dementia in a postmodern society, where new forms of narrative and, indeed, life seemingly become the norm. Like Richard Taylor, whom Helga Rohra had met at a conference, the

---

[47] For details, see the account by Assauer's daughter: Bettina Michel with Eva Mohr, *Papa, ich bin für Dich da. Wie Sie Demenzkranken helfen können* [Dad, I am there for you. How you can help dementia patients] (Munich: mvg Verlag, 2014), esp. pp. 154–161 (Michel 2014).

[48] See, e.g., Katrin Elger, 'Das Demenz-Dilemma' [The dementia dilemma], *Der Spiegel*, 19 September 2011 (Elger 2011); Amina Linke, 'Münchnerin (59): So lebe ich mit Demenz' [Citizen of Munich (59): this is how I live with dementia], *Münchner Abendzeitung*, 25 May 2012 (Linke 2012); Ulrike Luthmer-Lechner, 'Ich bin dement – na und?' [I am demented – so what?], *Göppinger Kreisnachrichten*, 14 March 2013 (Luthmer-Lechner 2013); and the interview with Michael Krons in the TV show 'Im Dialog' [In dialogue] on 17 February 2012; see: 'Helga Rohra – Im Dialog vom 17.02.2012', http://www.youtube.com/watch?v=Bq6M_3uCqQQ (accessed August 2016).

translator advocates an enabling dementia discourse, and acknowledges 'her friend Christine Bryden for the good exchange of ideas' (120). Building on this support, Rohra combines Taylor's teaching approach with Bryden's and Couturier's honesty, to lament that 'dementia is always considered from its end' (93). In this respect, Rohra's account reveals a change in patient discourse and activism. Patients have become more organised in terms of administrative infrastructure, and their writing is increasingly building on the narratives of those who succeeded in blazing a trail for postmodern self-representation.

Open Access This chapter is distributed under the terms of the Creative Commons Attribution 4.0 International License (http://creativecommons.org/licenses/by/4.0/), which permits use, duplication, adaptation, distribution and reproduction in any medium or format, as long as you give appropriate credit to the original author(s) and the source, a link is provided to the Creative Commons license and any changes made are indicated.

The images or other third party material in this chapter are included in the work's Creative Commons license, unless indicated otherwise in the credit line; if such material is not included in the work's Creative Commons license and the respective action is not permitted by statutory regulation, users will need to obtain permission from the license holder to duplicate, adapt or reproduce the material.

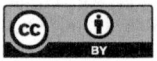

CHAPTER 6

Conclusion

Dementia Narratives: Shifter of Perspectives and Values

Abstract The conclusion considers the changes both caregiver and patient life-writing have gone through over a thirty-year period. It identifies these changes in a multilanguage approach as, partly, conditioned by the rising number of individuals with dementia and the increasing societal presence of the disease. At the same time, these changes have propelled forward a patient-centred development. More and more patients aim actively to participate in shaping the mainstream dementia discourse, which especially involves shifting notions of selfhood. A deliberation on very recent third-person caregiver narratives, including a graphic novel and a film documentary, highlights that this evolution in patient perception has reached broader societal levels, and promises to shift values in healthcare planning and socio-economic as well as cultural approaches to the condition.

Keywords Discourse changes · Film · Graphic memoir · Illness experience · Political patient

Es heißt, jede Erzählung sei eine Generalprobe für den Tod, denn jede Erzählung muss an ein Ende gelangen. Gleichzeitig bringt das Erzählen dadurch, dass es sich dem Verschwinden widmet, die verschwundenen Dinge zurück.

[It is said that every narrative is a dress rehearsal for death, because every narrative has to reach an end. At the same time, narrative brings back what has disappeared, because it is dedicated to disappearance.][1]

Illness is like old age in the way it relentlessly marginalizes its sufferers, transforming them from participants into spectators.[2]

Together with DSS, Helga Rohra and Christian Zimmermann have helped to instigate changes in the Alzheimer's disease patient discourse in Germany, just as the narratives by Richard Taylor, Christine Bryden and others are witness to global changes. These developments are equally manifest in caregiver accounts, whose portrayals reflect – like Arno Geiger's, Phillip Toledano's or Judith Fox's – conviction of the patient's continued identity and self. That such representations are more likely found in stories by male caregivers is partly related to their author-narrators' 'care-free' distance. That said, more recent narratives by female adult-child caregivers like Sally Magnusson or Donatella Di Pietrantonio similarly affirm the patient's continued identity by, for example, directly addressing the patient throughout in the second person; Di Pietrantonio indeed referring, like Toledano, to her mother as a river.[3]

Developments that demand more caregiver support and patient affirmation continue, also against the persistent numeric imbalance between caregiver and patient narratives. With Helga Rohra's powerful political statement in mind, I will close with two recent caregiver texts. I will illustrate how much and how quickly changes in discourse are now taking place, and how much potential there is for future change, both in the field of caregiving and in the appreciation of patient autonomy, even if there is the strong awareness of the patient's eventual dissolution. Alzheimer's disease

---

[1] Geiger, *Der alte König in seinem Exil*, p. 175 (Geiger 2011).

[2] Hadas, *Strange Relation*, p. 38 (Hadas 2011).

[3] Donatella Di Pietrantonio, *Mia madre è un fiume* [My mother is a river] (Rome: Elliot Edizioni S. R. L., 2010) (Di Pietrantonio 2010); Sally Magnusson, *Where Memories Go. Why Dementia Changes Everything* (London: Two Roads, 2014) (Magnusson 2014); on Di Pietrantonio's narrative, see also: Wilkinson, 'Remembering forgetting' (Wilkinson 2014).

has become – next to representing harsh biomedical facts – a synonym for caregiver burden, patient concerns and societal fears of aging and dependence. Therefore, allusions suffice to convey truths relating to the dementia experience. My reading of Sarah Leavitt's graphic memoir and David Sieveking's book and contemporaneously released cinematic documentary argues that, although the themes and needs in the context of dementia remain the same, the condition's presentation has become less forgiving, more aggressive, direct and honest than before.[4]

Alzheimer's Disease Narratives Today: New Media, Germane Stories

Reminiscent of Annie Ernaux's difficulties to locate and define herself in the imminent absence of her mother, Sarah Leavitt initially works through her experience of the mother's losses in short prose:

> She lost the concept of mother and daughter. She stopped saying my name. She asked me who I was. She did not respond at all when I entered the room. These were all deaths, weren't they? Or one long, slow death.[5]

Eventually, this Vancouver editor, writer and cartoonist depicts the 'cruel, relentless progression of losses' in a graphic memoir.[6] Yet, reminiscent of narratives by other adult-child caregivers, Leavitt obviously wanted to show 'the ways in which parts of her [mother Midge] endured' (7). She draws Midge's face with constancy for most of the narrative, with only her body posture signalling weakness, like Hank Spohr's stooping throughout the

---

[4] A recent analysis of fictional narratives addresses 'contradictions and systemic violence of our current culture of care'; I have not discovered life-writing texts that admit to abuse in dementia care relationships, even though caregiver burnout becomes more and more prominent; see: Lucy Burke, 'On (not) caring: tracing the meanings of care in the imaginative literature of the "Alzheimer's epidemic"', in *The Edinburgh Companion to the Critical Medical Humanities*, ed. by Anne Whitehead and Angela Woods (Edinburgh: Edinburgh University Press, 2016), pp. 596–610, p. 607 (Burke 2016).

[5] Sarah Leavitt, 'Kaddish', in *Beyond Forgetting. Poetry and Prose about Alzheimer's Disease*, ed. by Holly J. Hughes (Kent: The Kent State University Press, 2009), pp. 167–168, p. 167 (Leavitt 2009).

[6] Sarah Leavitt, *Tangles. A Story about Alzheimer's, My Mother, and Me* (London: Jonathan Cape, 2011), p. 7 (Leavitt 2011); all further references incorporated in the text.

narrative: her hands are raised and folded in front of her chest, suggesting an intimidated individual's gesture of protection.⁷ Near the end, two nasolabial lines carve out Midge's emaciation (118), and in her dying just one line contours her face, rendering her ghostlike (119) and, eventually, giving way to a black shadow (120).

Set against this decline, Leavitt ends this series with the reproduction of an actual drawing of her mother, prepared at the death bed (123). This choice highlights, together with copies of several of the mother's scribbled notes, the diary-like nature of Leavitt's narrative and her attempt to create:

> this book to remember her as she was before she got sick, but also to remember her as she was during her illness, [...] pieced together from my memories, my notes, and my sketches [...]: the tangled story of my mother, and me, and Alzheimer's. (7)

Yet, Leavitt arranges the comic's rectangles very systematically, hardly interrupting them in their size, as if they should bring order into her jumbled notes – and the mother's mind. Leavitt's partner describes Midge's mind as 'the garden this summer [...]. Tangled, but with spots of brightness', and Leavitt herself frames this with a wild arrangement of grass and flowers, a snail, and, difficult to identify, a dead animal (114).

Such attention to detail and allusion to despair and decline are characteristic of Leavitt's presentation, in which dark spaces and black/white inversion become particularly meaningful. Leavitt describes herself as inspired by work 'capturing gesture, focusing on the energy of the pose more than the details of the anatomy'.⁸ In this spirit, her drawings are reduced, and reduce, to the essential, forcing us to appreciate the raw upset of the diagnosis and its implications: Midge's insight 'I have Alzheimer's' (25), in white print on black, does not leave room for hope, just as the blackness engulfing the sad-looking mother does not leave any breathing space.

This speechless emptiness lends itself to a powerful depiction of the caregiver's loneliness in the medical discourse, which Leavitt continues to perceive as dominant and isolating, even after twenty-five years of caregiver agency and politically motivated writing. Three small black figures – mother,

---

⁷ Pease and Pease, *Body Language*, e.g., p. 99 (Pease and Pease 2005).

⁸ 'Reading guide. *Tangles*. Sarah Leavitt', http://www.freehand-books.com/wp-content/uploads/2012/03/Tangles-Reading-Guide.pdf (accessed December 2016).

father and daughter – are depicted in a vast empty space in front of the closed door to the doctor's office (35). The doctor himself is distant from both patient and caregivers, behind his barrier-like desk, and the interview situation leaves the hunched-up mother surrounded by assessment questions that are forced upon her in bold print (36).

Just as Judith Fox could build on the societal awareness of the condition's implications, Leavitt's narrative thrives on all she can draw, without having to comment on it, anymore and any further. A single-panel page shows the mother lonely and reduced (since covering just about ten percent of the page), with her back towards the onlooker; she only wears a top and underpants, with her trousers around her ankles (81). Likewise, the father, in his need of relief from the daily burden of caregiving and 'desperate for freedom', is shown as completely wrapped in a rope, with just his yelling mouth and splayed hands sticking out (117).

Leavitt's mercilessly honest presentation is certainly enabled by the narrative's graphic form, not least, since, as Ian Williams claims, autobiographical comics 'come from a radical background that respects self-publishing and small scale circulation'; and in requiring narrative brevity, the comic's disarming pictorial openness is complemented by textual directness rather than figurative language.[9] For example, Leavitt can write without the reservation suggested in the use of the child metaphor in Annie Ernaux's and other earlier narratives, bringing the truth about her mother's bathing to the point as follows:

> Mom's clothes were piled on the floor. There was dried shit in her underwear. The bathwater was full of small disintegrating bits of it. She was dipping her washcloth in the water and rubbing it over her skin. She had no sense of smell, true. But she could see. She just couldn't recognize. Couldn't recognize shit, dirt, shame. (60)

Leavitt lives, like Konek, at a distance from her parents, but comes home more and more often to share time with her mother, and eventually takes on caring for her. Yet, she 'couldn't do the work I'd brought with me to Fredericton' (73), and admits that she 'was sick of trying to fill in

---

[9] Ian Williams, 'Graphic medicine: how comics are revolutionizing the representation of illness', *Hektoen International. A Journal of Medical Humanities*, 3 (2012), http://www.hektoeninternational.org/index.php?option=com_content&view=article&id=353:graphic-medicine&catid=93&Itemid=716 (accessed August 2016) (Williams 2012).

the gaps in her speech. I was sick of helping her. I was sick of her being sick' (73). This anaphora illuminates Leavitt's speechlessness in the confrontation with her mother's condition. We may empathise with her frankness even more, when reading what the graphic presentation suggests to be taken from her diary entries: 'It gets hard to see someone as a person when they've become a list of needs: BATH, CLOTHES, BRUSH TEETH, WALK, FOOD, ETC' (85; emphasis original).

As such, *Tangles* is, as its subtitle suggests, Leavitt's story as much as it is her mother's, especially since Leavitt felt that '[a]s my mother changed, I changed too, forced to reconsider my own identity as a daughter and as an adult and to recreate my relationship with my mother' (7). Leavitt's memoir becomes the space, in which she can come to terms with herself and her coming out. And her narrative gains further meaning, because it deals with the added complication of providing dementia care in a heterosexist environment, when Leavitt, for example, openly writes:

> I could never have trimmed Mom's pubic hair. I never touched her between the legs without toilet paper or a washcloth between us. /I believe this was partly because I had touched women's bodies for sex, and because sometimes I feared being accused of perversion because of it. That all added to the weirdness of bathing and grooming my own mother in the first place. (111)

Leavitt does not make her sexual orientation a central topic, even though her being confronted with preconceptions against 'dykes' is alluded to throughout her drawings. Much rather, her narrative opens the discussion and awareness that service providers should 'begin to critically consider their attitudes and responses to carers whose social identities are increasingly diverse', because the caregiver's experience does, as we have seen, strongly impact on their relationship with the people they look after.[10] This analysis echoes Benjamin Fraser's exploration of a father's graphic narrative about his daughter María with autism. Fraser perceives of the author-narrator's self-representation as radically enabling, because it helps him to externalise:

---

[10] Elizabeth Price, 'Coming out to care: gay and lesbian carers' experiences of dementia services', *Health and Social Care in the Community*, 18 (2010), pp. 160–168, p. 167 (Price 2010); Angela M. Barbara, Sara A. Quandt and Roger T. Anderson, 'Experiences of lesbians in the health care environment', *Women and Health*, 34 (2001), pp. 45–62 (Barbara et al. 2001).

both his own frustrations with the social situations that surround disability and his love for his daughter, and in the process he also gives voice (or better, shape) to María's own struggles, joys, and ways of thinking in ways that only a parent might be able to do.[11]

A graphic narrative is more than a one-dimensional text that necessarily forces 'one view' on the reader, or a photograph, of which we assume that it depicts reality. A comic shows, as Douglas Wolk points out, 'things and people, real or imagined, moving in space and changing over time, as transformed through somebody's eye and hand'.[12] We can, in fact, read Leavitt's pictures as Midge's story of her illness. We can also read it as Leavitt's confrontation with, as well as her interpretation of, that story. In its two-dimensionality, a graphic memoir offers both: direct confrontation *and* personal perspective. Seen in this light, Leavitt's narrative is doubly personal and political, as it challenges onlookers to question their reaction to small detail and, thus, enforces their search for the larger truths. Its many black and white panels, like Phillip Toledano's white pages, open space and time for the viewer to work through Leavitt's agenda, and the large, quadratic picture book format etches its contents into our memory: actively to participate in the negotiation of a new sociopolitical dementia discourse.

Just as Leavitt opens new ways of looking at caregiving and broaching caregiver concerns that only recently have attracted attention, David Sieveking explores a new medium and perspective in filming his mother's dementia. Exhausted from daily caregiving, Sieveking's father Malte is in need of a holiday, and David is ready to look after his mother Margarete (Gretel) for two weeks. Departing from this initial constellation, filmmaker Sieveking and his friend, cinematographer Adrian Stähli, follow the family over a period of eighteen months, the collected material eventually yielding a ninety-minute motion picture.[13]

---

[11] Benjamin Fraser, *Disability Studies and Spanish Culture. Films, Novels, the Comic and the Public Exhibition* (Liverpool: Liverpool University Press, 2013), esp. Chap. 2, p. 39 (Fraser 2013).
[12] Douglas Wolk, *Reading Comics. How Graphic Novels Work and What They Mean* (Cambridge: Da Capo Press, 2007), p. 118 (Wolk 2007); consider also Susan Sontag's deliberations on how we read photographs, in *Regarding the Pain of Others* (Sontag 2004).
[13] David Sieveking, *Vergiss Mein Nicht. Wie meine Mutter ihr Gedächtnis verlor und meine Eltern die Liebe neu entdeckten* [Forget me not. How my mother lost her memory and my

Charges regarding the moral impropriety of publicly showing the mother's decay followed. For example, Rainer Erlinger questioned Malte Sieveking's reading out of some of his wife's diary entries, without Gretel being actually aware of this breach of confidentiality.[14] Similarly, a scene one third into the picture was debated at a public viewing, because Sieveking exposed his mother's weakness.[15] In this scene, Sieveking takes his mother to the local swimming pool (29:40), encouraging her to join him in the water, even though she continues to claim: 'Ich kann nicht mehr' [I cannot anymore; 30:07–30:14]. Gretel eventually trudges away from the pool, begging, the camera closing up on her face, 'können wir irgendwo hinsitzen, wo wir nicht sterben' [can we sit down somewhere, where we won't die; 30:58]. Pressured on this scene, Sieveking discloses that the attendant had wanted to arrest him, once aware that the scene was being filmed. However, the son further reveals that he had encouraged his mother so much, because she had truly enjoyed a swim several weeks earlier. His admitting to have 'too fervently tried to revive what had been before', lets us appreciate Sieveking's personal investment underlying the making of this film, which he intended to become a 'Denkmal für die Mutter' [memorial for the mother].[16]

This memory-making intention resonates with the meaning Konek, Geiger or Lindbergh assign to their narratives, and is captured in the leitmotif used in the marketing of the film. In reference to the opening scene that quickly zooms in on a wall of Gretel's Post-it® notes, accompanied by Sieveking's voiceover that 'at some point, I noticed all my mother's notes' (01:06–01:12), the film poster as well as DVD cover and menu incorporate this Post-it® motif. This strategy highlights the film as a space for creating memory, while equally emphasising the erosion of memory in Alzheimer's disease. One note reads: 'DAVID ist mein

---

parents rediscovered their love] (Farbfilm Verleih, 2012); released 31 January 2013 (Sieveking 2012).
[14] Rainer Erlinger, 'Vorgeführt im Verfall' [Exhibited in decay], *Süddeutsche Zeitung*, 5 February 2013 (Erlinger 2013).
[15] 'Potsdamer Filmgespräch. *Vergiss Mein Nicht*' [Potsdam film conversation. Forget me not], 19 March 2013, http://www.kreatives-brandenburg.de/veranstaltung/potsdamer-filmgesprach-vergiss-mein-nicht/ (accessed August 2016).
[16] Potsdam film conversation with the film and theatre director Andreas Dresen; available as bonus material on the DVD released by Farbfilm Home Entertainment (13:44; 05:26).

Jüngster und dreht einen Film über mich' [DAVID is my youngest and is shooting a film about me; emphasis original].[17]

That the cover of his eponymous book, which preceded the film release by three weeks, does not explore this Post-it® motif underscores Sieveking's understanding of the complementary purpose of his textual narrative; an interpretation supported by the book's slightly differing subtitle.[18] The book, like I discussed in relation to Thomas DeBaggio's text, embodies the note itself. Indeed, I take the timely coordinated publication of book and film as the key to Sieveking's mindful contribution to shifting the societal dementia discourse. In supplementing what a motion picture aimed at a broad audience cannot and should not show, the book offers contextual background, while also conveying an ethical and political framework for the film.

Like other caregiver narratives, the text's first half details the long path to Gretel's diagnosis, and her shrinking 'zu einem Schatten ihrer alten Persönlichkeit' [to the mere shadow of her old personality; 67], and leads up to the time span depicted in the film. The documentary ends some time before Gretel is admitted to hospital. Her actual time in the hospital ('Krankenhaus') is recounted in the book's second half. Sieveking's play on words 'Im kranken Haus' [In the sick house; 142] anticipates the family's grappling with questions regarding end-of-life care, as Thomas Graboys had broached them, and highlights insufficient support from healthcare staff. Likewise, the chapter on an 'Irrtum zweiter Klasse' [Error of the second class; 161] openly denounces the money-related quality of attention patients receive in the German healthcare system.

Anticipating the ethical issues relating to the film's production, Sieveking freely admits that 'Gretel looked less advantageous for the camera' (155), once she was in hospital.[19] But in view of his mother's

---

[17] Fraser similarly comments on the use of a specific narrative motif, namely a set of drawers, in the DVD menu and first screen image of a film based on a comic book; see: Fraser, *Disability Studies and Spanish Culture*, p. 59 (Fraser 2013).

[18] David Sieveking, *Vergiss Mein Nicht. Wie meine Mutter ihr Gedächtnis verlor und ich meine Eltern neu entdeckte* [Forget me not. How my mother lost her memory and I discovered my parents anew] (Freiburg im Breisgau: Herder, 2013) (Sieveking 2013); references incorporated in the text; released 9 January 2013.

[19] See also the conversation between David Sieveking and the film's producer Martin Heisler in the context of the German film prize 2013, inter alia, about marketing issues; available as part of bonus material on the DVD released by Farbfilm Home Entertainment (7:05–7:41).

rapid deterioration and nearing death, he ponders, reminiscent of Arno Geiger's reflections, how to let the film come to an end: 'to leave it as it is, simply ignoring the last phase in Gretel's life or just mentioning it with a text, does not seem correct' (210). Eventually, he opens the film again, after cutting was already completed, to add a final scene 'six months later' (84:06), once Gretel has returned home from the hospital. In this scene, Mrs. Sieveking rests on a highly functional hospital bed, surrounded by children and grandchildren (84:15–85:25). The camera captures Gretel's face smiling as she takes in her husband's nearness for almost half a minute (84:58–85:25), before the screen darkens and text appears which dedicates the film to her, listing her date of birth and death.

While Margarete Sieveking's emaciated face and slow movements encapsulate all that Sieveking had 'not wanted to document with the camera' (210), this scene adds to the viewer's deliberations on patient dignity, spousal duties and the quality of end-of-life care. Film and book push this discussion even further, because filming per se reveals itself as caregiving, if not therapy, as Sieveking remarks:

> In der Gegenwart von Kamera-, Tonmann und mir, drei jungen Männern, die sich stark für sie interessierten, blühte meine Mutter richtiggehend auf. 'Die beste Therapie für Gretel sind David und der Film!', fand mein Vater.
>
> [In the presence of camera, soundman and myself, three young men, who were very much interested in her, my mother really blossomed. My father found that 'the best therapy for Gretel are David and the film!'; 16].

The one question that then returns again and again in reflections on caregiver life-writing is, as Erlinger mentions in his film review, whether these narratives make the patients into Alzheimer's disease 'victims'; whether, as seen in Walter Jens's case, they do not leave any space for the recognition of their achievements and continued memory, while, in the present case, helping Sieveking in his career development. I want to consider this question by looking back to similar accusations made against John Bayley. Bayley retorted that his wife had given herself to science in consenting to a study carried out on her linguistic abilities in correlation to her brain atrophy.[20] Murdoch actively worked for the cause of dementia, aware of the power of her own prominence. Similarly, Sieveking and his

---

[20] Garrard et al., 'The effects of very early Alzheimer's disease' (Garrard et al. 2005).

family perceive the showing of this film as a continuation of Margarete Sieveking's political commitment. For Bayley, Murdoch's memory as a writer will continue alongside of these efforts, since, as the scholar consoles himself, '[h]er genius lives in her books' (560), 'Iris's books live on' (582); she is 'memories, images in the mind, words in books' (631). Sieveking offers a testament to his mother that gives the cinemagoer the feeling that dementia can leave the patient, like Helga Rohra, smiling, and the caregiver aware of her continued presence.

Also, the film appears as 'an open journey', exposing dementia as a condition of spontaneity and continued potential.[21] The story's twists and turns which eventually pitch it to a wider audience are initiated by Mrs. Sieveking herself. She unexpectedly pulls her son out of the lethargic exhaustion of his first week of caregiving by asking: 'are you coming with me to Stuttgart' (33:21), her place of birth. It is this move that prompts Sieveking to look into his mother's past, and contributes to the film being blended with black and white photographs as well as short scenes from old film recordings. These documents highlight Gretel Sieveking's activities in a radical socialist student organisation during the late 1960s. Their arrangement as part of the film about the mother's illness underscores Sieveking's emphasis on the mother's activity in the present as building on her pursuits in the past; a conceptualisation that distances Sieveking's motion picture from Grothé's uni-dimensional photographic series. That Sieveking concomitantly discovers that his parents had led an open marriage further appeals to the cinemagoer's desire for a happy closure and outlook: Sieveking can document a positive effect on Malte of caregiving for his wife, in that it makes him realise that 'she did not receive the love she deserved' (221). At the very same time, this relationship storyline challenges the general public as well as the medico-clinical researcher to reconsider their conceptualisation of the condition as one of decline and loss alone.[22]

---

[21] Potsdam film conversation (04:24), see p. 124 fn. 16.

[22] Conference 'Im Fokus: Menschen mit Demenz – Wenn Praxis und Forschung verbunden werden' [In focus: people with dementia – when practice and research are being linked], University Heidelberg, 18 April 2013, http://www.nar.uni-heidelberg.de/veranstaltun gen/kongress/archiv.html (accessed October 2016); the conference was organised in the framework of the graduate training programme 'Demenz' [dementia] aimed at 'improving health care quality and structures'; Sieveking's film and its discussion with the public – led by

STORIES OF DEMENTIA: PEDAGOGICAL, POLITICAL, REPRESENTATIVE

Writing the story of one's own illness, or that of the parent or spouse, is usually aimed at offering an alternative to the culturally dominant narrative regarding that illness.[23] I set out to consider every available book-length patient-authored text. But at the same time, the present analysis had to fall back on a small selection of many caregiver memoirs, the choice of which, I am fully aware, represents a political act in itself. The numeric imbalance between caregiver-authored third-person accounts and patient-authored first-person narratives on the book market easily furthers sociocultural preconception of patients as being unable to narrate their story and, therefore, unaware of themselves as individuals. This passive stereotype is then further enhanced by caregivers, who place, under the impression of the patient's accelerated aging and increasing need for help with daily chores, questions as to their own identity and future into the centre of their story. Additionally, narrators who feel particularly exposed to the stress and strain of caregiving for patients in advanced stages of the condition understandably tend to report the relative as both cause and object of their burden.

It is the patients' fear of this loss of recognition and standing within their social environment and, thus, their identity in the later stages of their condition (when others unavoidably write about them) that brings them in the early stages of their illness to challenge such reification. Indeed, they persuasively emphasise their agency by speaking from a position that purportedly precludes narration from the first-person perspective, and by choosing narrative forms that conjecture control of the illness process.[24] Their emotional urgency, in turn, becomes – as G. Thomas Couser observes in his analysis of breast cancer and HIV/AIDS memoirs – most apparent from the time delay between the composition of their narrative and its consumption, as it harshly dismantles their 'tale'.[25] Likewise, the stark

---

the programme's initiators Konrad Beyreuther, molecular biologist, and Andreas Kruse, gerontologist – closed the symposium.

[23] Couser, *Recovering Bodies* (Couser 1997); Hawkins, *Reconstructing Illness* (Hawkins 1999).

[24] Burke, 'Alzheimer's disease', p. 1 (Burke 2007).

[25] I am taking this term from Jeffrey Aronson, 'Autopathography: the patient's tale' (Aronson 2000).

difference in meaning that patients as compared to caregivers impose on images, and the lack of successful formulation, for example, of their illness as journey highlight their struggle to assert themselves in a condition that increasingly compromises their independence.

Set against these considerations, the powerful pictures drawn by relatives, who perceive of themselves as partner rather than sole nurturer or consider the condition as integral to aging, match patients' self-portrayals and identity-affirming needs. Nevertheless, even in enabling presentations and personal constellations where caregivers can create opportunities for quality time with their relative, helplessness and feelings of guilt remain, as Reeve Lindbergh points out:

> In a situation like mine, there is memory, and there is frustration, and there is grief, and there is guilt. In fact, there is more guilt than anything else. No matter how good the care provided, no matter how much attention or how much money is spent to address their needs, no matter how extensive the medical treatment lavished upon our beloved elders, there is always guilt, and it is always the same. (24)

Ultimately, both patient and caregiver do, despite their different agendas, follow the urge to draw continuity, where memory loss, increasing dependence and nearing death destroy coherence. Considered from this angle, I agree with John Wiltshire that the confrontation with Alzheimer's disease condenses all illness experience most acutely, and a narrative about dementia perhaps offers the fullest view of what it means to be ill. Rita Charon has summarised this possibility for Rachel Hadas's narrative, which also particularly centres on feelings of guilt in relation to the husband's placement:

> While *Strange Relation* relates one illness and the life of one family, it is also, poetically, about all illnesses, all families, all struggles, all living. The art achieves the dual life of the universal and the particular, marking it as timeless, making it for us all necessary.[26]

---

[26] Charon's praise for Hadas's narrative; see: Hadas, *Strange Relation*, p. i (Hadas 2011).

As Alzheimer's disease embodies the loss of personhood, writing about it becomes a searching for meaning-making substitutes, where metaphorical language turns into expressions and assertions of the self as much as the narrative itself.[27] As Arno Geiger tells us in the quote offered at the beginning of this chapter, the confrontation with death brings narratives by patients and caregivers together. The title of this work anticipated it: dementia narratives are a form of *life*-writing. The condition is perceived as threatening the mind and, thus, personal identity with such intensity that it cannot simply remain a crisis and, thus, a chapter within (the musings on) a life.[28] Instead, it must become the central focus of a narrative that explores the full existential implications of the condition and asserts that cognitive abilities and consciousness are not the lone identifiers of a person.

In the light of the ever-aging population, Alzheimer's disease is the most feared neurological condition today; and it may remain so for several more decades, given that a complete understanding of its cause continues to be elusive and its treatment therefore only symptom-based and, currently, of limited efficacy. This book has explored how individuals affected by the condition – caregivers as well as individuals with dementia themselves – engage with and aspire to shape the culturally dominant dementia narrative. It has done so by reading their narratives against what have become Health Humanities canonical texts, only alluding to psychoanalytical and phenomenological implications for example in the context of sons' life-writing.[29] One of the core aims of this study was to amplify the voices of those whose texts it critiqued. As such, the discussion has concentrated on the immediate relevance for policy changes and healthcare approaches of the author-narrators' poetic choices and political concerns. Concurrently, it has become clear that their intentions and needs have shifted over the thirty-year period covered in this analysis, raising perhaps the question as to a more expansive chronological contextualisation of these

---

[27] James Olney, *Metaphors of Self. The Meaning of Autobiography* (Princeton: Princeton University Press, 1972), pp. 34–35 (Olney 1972).

[28] See also: Couser, *Recovering Bodies*, pp. 6, 14 (Couser 1997).

[29] These theoretical paradigms are anticipated to gain renewed relevance for the analysis of lived experience; see: Neil Vickers, 'Illness narratives', in *A History of English Autobiography*, ed. by Adam Smyth (New York: Cambridge University Press, 2016), pp. 388–401 (Vickers 2016).

developments, not least given the historical timings of the studies, for example, by Wiltshire, Woodward and Cohen.

What this book, for example, could not do in its space and scope is more fully to consider the historical grounding of frequently reifying and infantilising patient presentations. Thomas DeBaggio's first narrative, for instance, negotiates with the recent scientific dementia discourse to an extent that invites a deeper reflection on changes in this discourse since the condition's inception in medico-scientific terms in the 1880s.[30] Taking then into account the power-shifting effects of life-writing discussed in this book, it is not unlikely that these developments impact also on how scientific researchers and practicing clinicians have approached the condition over time. I am addressing the dynamics between scientific, medical and literary renderings of dementia across such an extended timespan in future work, also in the light of recent observations regarding shifting notions of memory and forgetting.[31]

Also shifting notions of aging over an extended timespan will further illuminate the claims made in this book, whose focus remained on what is usually referred to as the Western world. But population aging and age-related cognitive decline also increasingly challenge economies like China, India and South Asia, and this book's multilanguage approach suggests that its insights likely expand to other cultures. Most of all, these insights demand that the patient's continued identity – as also being more and more dependent on the caregiver's support (and eventually necessary presentation) and society's perception – become the mainstream Alzheimer's disease narrative. This is especially so, since, as Nortin Hadler emphasises:

> Aging is not a disease, and frail elderly persons are not a burden. Aging is a privilege of life in a resource-advantaged society, and the elderly, including frail elderly persons, enrich that society.[32]

In the awareness of the little time available to them, both patients and caregivers draw energy and help from their act of writing. This very writing

---

[30] Zimmermann, 'Alzheimer's disease metaphors' (Zimmermann forthcoming).

[31] Jens Brockmeier, *Beyond the Archive. Memory, Narrative, and the Autobiographical Process* (New York: Oxford University Press, 2015) (Brockmeier 2015).

[32] Nortin M. Hadler, *Rethinking Aging. Growing Old and Living Well in an Overtreated Society* (Chapel Hill: The University of North Carolina Press, 2011), p. 172 (Hadler 2011).

becomes their and the reader's opportunity to bring about healing through the changes that society should realise in learning from such writing. Giving such narratives increasing attention and using them for educational and training purposes will sharpen society's eyes for disabling and belittling misrepresentations, and pave the way for thoughtful transformations in the perception of dementia and its sufferers.[33] These transformations will impact on the ethical and socio-economic consequences of our dealing with an aging population; they will influence a committed alleviation of carer burden through social support systems and altered healthcare policies; they will modify sociocultural attitudes towards early-stage demented patients; and they will frame a more considerate care for patients with advanced conditions.

---

[33] See also: Hannah Zeilig, 'The critical use of narrative and literature in gerontology', *International Journal of Ageing and Later Life*, 6.2 (2011), pp. 7–37 (Zeilig 2011).

Open Access This chapter is distributed under the terms of the Creative Commons Attribution 4.0 International License (http://creativecommons.org/licenses/by/4.0/), which permits use, duplication, adaptation, distribution and reproduction in any medium or format, as long as you give appropriate credit to the original author(s) and the source, a link is provided to the Creative Commons license and any changes made are indicated.

The images or other third party material in this chapter are included in the work's Creative Commons license, unless indicated otherwise in the credit line; if such material is not included in the work's Creative Commons license and the respective action is not permitted by statutory regulation, users will need to obtain permission from the license holder to duplicate, adapt or reproduce the material.

Bibliography of Dementia Narratives

The following list gives an overview of the narratives referred to in this book by date of publication. The aim is to help orient the reader with a synopsis that offers key information on the narratives discussed in detail in the text (marked with an asterisk).

Caregiver Narratives

1982
Inoue, Yasushi, *Chronicle of My Mother*

1983
Roach, Marion, 'Another Name for Madness'

1991
* Ernaux, Annie, *A Woman's Story*
  A French daughter's narrative of her mother's life story; composed and published after the mother's death (and discussed in conjunction with her diary; see below 1999).
* Konek, Carol Wolfe, *Daddyboy. A Family's Struggle with Alzheimer's*
  An American daughter's narrative of her father, exploring the daughter–father relationship; strong emphasis on the perceived continuity of the father's influence on and presence within the daughter's life; published after the father's death.

1993
Ignatieff, Michael, *Scar Tissue*
> Possibly fictional account by a Canadian son about his mother's dementia; strong emphasis on philosophical notions of memory loss.

1995
* Spohr, Betty Baker, with Jean Valens Bullard, *Catch a Falling Star. Living with Alzheimer's*
> The narrative of an American spouse caring for her husband; while published after the husband's death, the writing and drawing process accompanied the narrator throughout her living with the husband; a narrative of largely utilitarian character.

1996
Wall, Frank, *Where Did Mary Go? A Loving Husband's Struggle with Alzheimer's*
> Narrative by an American husband about his wife's dementia; very candid account of predominantly utilitarian character; published after the wife's death.

Zabbia, Kim Howes, *Painted Diaries. A Mother and Daughter's Experience through Alzheimer's*

1997
Davidson, Ann, *Alzheimer's. A Love Story. One Year in My Husband's Journey*
> Account by an American wife about her husband's illness; strong emphasis on the challenges of everyday life; published during the husband's lifetime.

1998
* Bayley, John, *Iris: A Memoir of Iris Murdoch*

Grant, Linda, *Remind Me Who I Am, Again*
> Narrative by a British daughter about her mother's vascular dementia; strong autobiographical notion.

1999
* Ernaux, Annie, *I Remain in Darkness*
> Diary entries by a French daughter, mostly made after frequent visits in the nursing home, where she observes the mother's losses and decline; published long after the mother's death and following the publication of her short biography (see above 1991).

Holroyd, Michael, *Basil Street Blues. A Family Story*

2000
Pierce, Charles P., *Hard to Forget. An Alzheimer's Story*

Zacharias, Sylvia, *Diagnose Alzheimer: Helmut Zacharias. Ein Bericht* [Diagnosis Alzheimer's: Helmut Zacharias. A report]
> Account by a German medical journalist about her father; endorsed by an organisation supporting medico-scientific research as well as patients and caregivers.

2001
Franzen, Jonathan, 'My Father's Brain'
* Lindbergh, Reeve, *No More Words. A Journal of My Mother, Anne Morrow Lindbergh*
   Narrative by the daughter of the American pilot and writer Anne Morrow Lindbergh, originating from notes and diary entries on the mother's illness, but published after the mother's death; strong emphasis on the mother's continued (though silent) presence.

2002
Laborde, Françoise, *Pourquoi ma mère me rend folle* [Why my mother drives me crazy]

2003
Bayley, John, *The Iris Trilogy*
Buades, Margarita Retuerto, *Mi vida junto a un enfermo de Alzheimer* [My life next to an Alzheimer's patient]
Laborde, Françoise, *Ma mère n'est pas un philodendron* [My mother is not a philodendron]

2006
* Appignanesi, Josh, *Ex Memoria. Some Memories Fade. Others Keep Returning*
   Autobiographically inspired short film about the elderly patient Eva, who experiences isolation and lacking awareness of her life history by both professional caregivers and her close family in a nursing home setting.

2007
* Grothé, Jean, *Alzheimer. Un journal photographique* [Alzheimer's. A photographic diary]
   A collection of photographs and short notes by a Canadian son, who accompanied his mother throughout the final three years of her illness; published after the mother's death; emphasis on the mother's seated portrayal.

2008
Wilhoit, Mary, *As She Was Dying. An Alzheimer's Journal*

2009
* Fox, Judith, *I Still Do. Loving and Living with Alzheimer's*
   Photo book by an American spouse about her husband, with strong emphasis on the continued partnership within and throughout the illness; the husband's awareness of the photos being taken is to be assumed.

Gillies, Andrea, *Keeper. Living with Nancy. A Journey into Alzheimer's*
   Narrative by a British daughter-in-law detailing her caregiving experience; published after the mother-in-law had been placed into a care home.

Jens, Inge, *Unvollständige Erinnerungen* [Incomplete memories]
   Autobiography of the German scholar, writer and editor that includes a chapter dedicated to her husband's condition.

* Jens, Tilman, *Demenz. Abschied von meinem Vater* [Dementia. Farewell to my father]
   A German journalist's memoir of the famous philologist father's illness; the narrative places strong emphasis on the patient's losses and potential national-socialist past, and was published while the father was still alive.

Rota, Nucci A., *La bimbamamma. Cosa vuol dire convivere con l'Alzheimer. Il diario di una figlia* [The mommy girl. What it means to share your life with Alzheimer's. A daughter's diary]
   Account by an Italian daughter about her mother's memory loss; detailed description of confrontation with isolating medical discourse; published after the mother's death.

2010

Di Pietrantonio, Donatella, *Mia madre è un fiume* [My mother is a river]

Jens, Tilman, *Vatermord. Wider einen Generalverdacht* [Patricide. Against a general suspicion]

* Toledano, Phillip, *Days with My Father*
   An Italo-American son's photographic memoir of his father; the photos are taken with the father's approval, and emphasise his humanity and continued personality within dementia; published after the father's death.

2011

* Geiger, Arno, *Der alte König in seinem Exil* [The old king in his exile]
   An Austrian writer's memoir of his father's life with dementia; strong emphasis on the father's continued personality and dignity within the condition; published while the father is still alive, with the ethical implications of this choice being discussed.

* Hadas, Rachel, *Strange Relation. A Memoir of Marriage, Dementia, and Poetry*
   Memoir by an American professor of English about her husband; strong emphasis on the perceived growing isolation within the relationship and the burden of the decision to place the husband into institutionalised care; published nine months before the patient's death.

* Leavitt, Sarah, *Tangles. A Story about Alzheimer's, My Mother, and Me*
   First graphic memoir by a Canadian daughter about her mother's illness; published after the mother's death; the candid presentation highlights the family's difficulties in coming to terms with caregiving for, and witnessing changes in, the female head of the family.

2013
* Sieveking, David, *Vergiss Mein Nicht. Wie meine Mutter ihr Gedächtnis verlor und meine Eltern die Liebe neu entdeckten* [Forget me not. How my mother lost her memory and my parents rediscovered their love]
    A German filmmaker's documentary about his mother's final eighteen months with dementia; exploration of the mother's past and the parents' relationship; in conjunction with the simultaneously published book offering important sociopolitical criticism.
Giovanna Venturino, *Il tuo mare di nulla. La mia mamma e l'Alzheimer* [Your sea of nothingness. My mother and Alzheimer's]

2014
Magnusson, Sally, *Where Memories Go. Why Dementia Changes Everything*
Michel, Bettina, with Eva Mohr, *Papa, ich bin für Dich da. Wie Sie Demenzkranken helfen können* [Dad, I am there for you. How you can help dementia patients]

PATIENT NARRATIVES

1989
* Davis, Robert, *My Journey into Alzheimer's Disease. Helpful Insights for Family and Friends. A True Story*
    The first patient-authored narrative by an American vicar; following the traditional journey myth, the narrative centres on the patient's Christian faith and acceptance of his illness; composed with the help of the patient's wife.

1993
* McGowin, Diana Friel, *Living in the Labyrinth. A Personal Journey through the Maze of Alzheimer's*
    The first patient-authored narrative that attracted international attention; the American narrative follows the traditional journey myth and acknowledges the husband's help in the epilogue.

1996
* Rose, Larry, *Show Me the Way to Go Home*
    American narrative that follows the journey myth; strong emphasis on continued activity within the condition, and criticism of insufficient societal support and acceptance of the illness (see also 2003).

1998
Boden, Christine, *Who Will I Be When I Die?*
* Henderson, Cary Smith, *Partial View. An Alzheimer's Journal*

Tape-recorded narrative snippets by an American professor of history; transcribed by his daughter, framed by the wife's introduction and complemented by a professional journalist's photos; narrative by a patient in the advanced stages of his illness.

2002
* DeBaggio, Thomas, *Losing My Mind. An Intimate Look at Life with Alzheimer's*
The first of two narratives by a journalist turned professional herb grower (see also 2003); the American author-narrator aims to depict the condition-related cognitive decline in the narrative's form; strong emphasis on perceived losses.

2003
* DeBaggio, Thomas, *When it Gets Dark. An Enlightened Reflection on Life with Alzheimer's*
The American patient's second narrative (see also 2002) aims to depict the condition-related cognitive decline just as his first text did, but the illness's progression is clearly noticed in the narrative's content and presentation.
* Lee, Jeanne L., *Just Love Me. My Life Turned Upside-Down by Alzheimer's*
An openly acknowledged professional writer structures the American patient's notes and tape recordings; strong emphasis on acceptance of the condition and continued capabilities within the illness.

Rose, Larry, *Larry's Way. Another Look at Alzheimer's from the Inside*

2004
* Couturier, Claude, *Puzzle. Journal d'une Alzheimer* [Jigsaw. Diary of an Alzheimer's patient]
I believe this to be the only available diary by an Alzheimer's disease patient; the French artist chronicles her experiences and difficulties in daily life, while emphasising her continued activism, long before publication was considered.

2005
* Bryden, Christine, *Dancing with Dementia. My Story of Living Positively with Dementia*
An Australian rebirth narrative based on Bryden's Alzheimer's diagnosis being corrected to that of frontotemporal dementia (see also 1998, Boden); challenging readers on their common conceptualisations of the condition; claiming patients' continued identity.

2006
Schneider, Charles, *Don't Bury Me, It Ain't Over Yet!*

2007
Mobley, Tracy, *Young Hope. The Broken Road*
* Taylor, Richard, *Alzheimer's from the Inside Out*
    A collection of short essays by an American psychologist, who aims to further a politically correct dementia discourse; issued with a healthcare publisher, his narrative purposefully supports the author's activism until his death in 2015.

2008
* Graboys, Thomas, with Peter Zheutlin, *Life in the Balance. A Physician's Memoir of Life, Love, and Loss with Parkinson's Disease and Dementia*
    The Harvard cardiologist suffers from Lewy body dementia; in collaboration with a professional writer, he describes the effects of the condition on his private and professional life; discussion of end-of-life choices.

2009
Donohue, Mike, *From AA to AD, a Wistful Travelogue*

2011
* Rohra, Helga, *Aus dem Schatten treten. Warum ich mich für unsere Rechte als Demenzbetroffene einsetze* [Stepping out of the shadow. Why I am advocating our rights as those afflicted by dementia]
    One of the first two narratives by German dementia patients; written with an assistant, this text authoritatively carves out the patient's continued identity and independence, and highlights personal and socio-economic struggles of early-onset patients.
Zimmermann, Christian, and Peter Wißmann, *Auf dem Weg mit Alzheimer. Wie sich mit einer Demenz leben lässt* [On the road with Alzheimer's. How it is possible to live with dementia]

2012
* Assauer, Rudi, *Wie ausgewechselt. Verblassende Erinnerungen an mein Leben* [Like substituted. Fading memories of my life]
    Based on numerous interviews, the narrative reveals itself as the biography of a football manager; interspersed with frequent text passages representing the patient's original quotes, the text remains largely focused on the patient's career as a sportsman.

WORKS CITED

Abraham, Ruth, *When Words Have Lost Their Meaning. Alzheimer's Patients Communicate through Art* (Westport: Praeger, 2005).
Almkvist, Ove, Neuropsychological features of early Alzheimer's disease: preclinical and clinical stages, *Acta Neurologica Scandinavica Supplementum*, 165 (1996), 63–71.
Alzheimer's Disease International, 'In memory of Richard Taylor'; http://www.alz.co.uk/news/in-memory-of-richard-taylor-phd (accessed August 2016).
'Alzheimer's research advocate Tom DeBaggio dies'; http://www.npr.org/2011/02/22/133971224/Alzheimers-Advocate-Thomas-DeBaggio-Dies (accessed August 2016).
Amanzio, Martina, Geminiani, Giuliano, Leotta, Daniela, and Stefano Cappa, Metaphor comprehension in Alzheimer's disease: novelty matters, *Brain and Language*, 107 (2008), 1–10.
Anderson, Linda, *Autobiography* (Abingdon: Routledge, 2001).
Appignanesi, Josh, *Ex Memoria. Some Memories Fade. Others Keep Returning* (Missing in Action Films Ltd., 2006).
Appignanesi, Josh, '*Ex Memoria*'; http://www.joshappignanesi.com/EX-MEMORIA (accessed August 2016).
Aronson, Jeffrey, Autopathography: the patient's tale, *Biomedical Journal*, 321 (2000), 1599–1602.
Aronson, Jeffrey, 'The patients' tales collection'; https://sites.google.com/a/patientstales.org/home/home (accessed August 2016).
Assauer, Rudi, *Wie ausgewechselt. Verblassende Erinnerungen an mein Leben* (Munich: Riva, 2012).

Baker, Kevin L., and Noelle Robertson, Coping with caring for someone with dementia: reviewing the literature about men, *Aging & Mental Health*, 12.4 (2008), 413–422.
Ballenger, Jesse F., *Self, Senility, and Alzheimer's Disease in Modern America. A History* (Baltimore: The Johns Hopkins University Press, 2006).
Banerjee, Sube, The macroeconomics of dementia – will the world economy get Alzheimer's disease? *Archives of Medical Research*, 43.8 (2012), 705–709.
Barbara, Angela M., Quandt, Sara A., and Roger T. Anderson, Experiences of lesbians in the health care environment, *Women and Health*, 34 (2001), 45–62.
Bartels, Emily C., Outside the box: surviving survival, *Literature and Medicine*, 28.2 (2009), 237–252.
Basting, Anne Davis, Looking back from loss: views of the self in Alzheimer's disease, *Journal of Aging Studies*, 17 (2003), 87–99.
Basting, Anne Davis, *Forget Memory. Creating Better Lives for People with Dementia* (Baltimore: The Johns Hopkins University Press, 2009).
Bayley, John, *The Iris Trilogy* (London: Abacus, 2003).
Bell, Chris, Is disability studies actually white disability studies?, In *The Disability Studies Reader, 3rd edition*, ed. by Lennard J. Davis (New York: Routledge, 2010), 374–382.
Bernlef, J., *Out of Mind*, trans. by Adrienne Dixon (London: Faber and Faber, 1988).
Boden, Christine, *Who Will I Be When I Die?* (Sydney: Harper Collins, 1998).
Boland, Anne, and Philippe Cappeliez, Optimism and neuroticism as predictors of coping and adaptation in older women, *Personality and Individual Differences*, 22.6 (1997), 909–919.
Boller, François, History of dementia, *Handbook of Clinical Neurology*, 89 (2008), 3–13.
Brandon, Valerie, 'Foreword' to Jeanne L. Lee, *Just Love Me. My Life Turned Upside-Down by Alzheimer's* (West Lafayette: Purdue University Press, 2003), xiv–xv.
Brockmeier, Jens, Questions of meaning: memory, dementia, and the post-autobiographical perspective, In *Beyond Loss: Dementia, Identity, Personhood*, ed. by Lars-Christer Hydén, Hilde Lindemann and Jens Brockmeier (New York: Oxford University Press, 2014), 69–90.
Brockmeier, Jens, *Beyond the Archive. Memory, Narrative, and the Autobiographical Process* (New York: Oxford University Press, 2015).
Brody, Howard, *Stories of Sickness, 2nd edition* (New York: Oxford University Press, 2003).
Bruner, Jerome, *Making Stories. Law, Literature, Life* (Cambridge: Harvard University Press, 2002).
Bryden, Christine, *Dancing with Dementia. My Story of Living Positively with Dementia* (London: Jessica Kingsley Publishers, 2005).
Buades, Margarita Retuerto, *Mi vida junto a un enfermo de Alzheimer* (Madrid: La Esfera de los Libros S. L., 2003).

Burack-Weiss, Ann, *The Caregiver's Tale. Loss and Renewal in Memoirs of Family Life* (New York: Columbia University Press, 2006).
Burke, Lucy, Introduction: thinking about cognitive impairment, *Journal of Literary Disability*, 2.1 (2008a), i–iv.
Burke, Lucy, 'The country of my disease': genes and genealogy in Alzheimer's life-writing, *Journal of Literary Disability*, 2.1 (2008b), 63–74.
Burke, Lucy, On (not) caring: tracing the meanings of care in the imaginative literature of the 'Alzheimer's epidemic', In *The Edinburgh Companion to the Critical Medical Humanities*, ed. by Anne Whitehead and Angela Woods (Edinburgh: Edinburgh University Press, 2016), 596–610.
Burke, Lucy, 'Alzheimer's disease: personhood and first person testimony', Presentation at the inaugural conference of the 'Cultural Disability Studies Research Network', Liverpool, May 2007; http://www.cdsrn.org.uk/Burke_CDSRN_2007.pdf (accessed August 2011); but no longer available.
Burkhardt, Ute, Lang, Dorothee, Mohr, Franziska, Schwarzkopf, Tina M., and Martina Zimmermann, Literature and science: a different look inside neurodegeneration, *Advances in Physiology Education*, 36 (2012), 68–71.
Burns, Alastair, The burden of Alzheimer's disease, *International Journal of Neuropsychopharmacology*, 3 (2000), S31–S38.
Bury, Michael, Chronic illness as biographical disruption, *Sociology of Health and Illness*, 4 (1982), 167–182.
Calasanti, Toni, and Mary E. Bowen, Spousal caregiving and crossing gender boundaries: maintaining gendered identities, *Journal of Aging Studies*, 20 (2006), 253–263.
Chappell, Neena L., and Valerie K. Kuehne, Congruence among husband and wife caregivers, *Journal of Aging Studies*, 12.3 (1998), 239–254.
Charazac, Pierre-Marie, Loss of identity in Alzheimer's disease: a psychoanalytic approach, *Psychologie et Neuropsychiatrie du Vieillissement*, 7.3 (2009), 169–174.
Charon, Rita, *Narrative Medicine. Honoring the Stories of Illness* (New York: Oxford University Press, 2006).
Chivers, Sally, *The Silvering Screen. Old Age and Disability in Cinema* (Toronto: University of Toronto Press, 2011).
Chow, Tiffany W., Personality in frontal lobe disorders, *Current Psychiatry Reports*, 2.5 (2000), 446–451.
'Christine Bryden. Dementia from an insider's perspective'; http://www.christinebryden.com/ (accessed August 2016).
Clarke, Charlotte L., Wilkinson, Heather, Keady, John, and Catherine E. Gibb, *Risk Assessment and Management for Living Well with Dementia* (London: Jessica Kingsley Publishers, 2011).
Cohen, Donna, and Carl Eisdorfer, *The Loss of Self: A Family Resource for the Care of Alzheimer's Disease and Related Disorders* (New York: W. W. Norton, 2002).

Cohen, Lawrence, *No Aging in India. Alzheimer's, the Bad Family, and Other Modern Things* (Berkeley: University of California Press, 1999).
Conway, Kathlyn, *Illness and the Limits of Expression* (Ann Arbor: The University of Michigan Press, 2007).
Couser, G. Thomas, *Recovering Bodies. Illness, Disability, and Life Writing* (Madison: The University of Wisconsin Press, 1997).
Couser, G. Thomas, Memoir and (lack of) memory: filial narratives of paternal dementia, In *New Essays on Life Writing and the Body*, ed. by Christopher Stuart and Stephanie Todd (Newcastle upon Tyne: Cambridge Scholars Publishing, 2009), 223–241; http://www.academia.edu/8298268/Memoir_and_Lack_of_Memory_Filial_Narratives_of_Paternal_Dementia (accessed August 2016).
Couturier, Claude, *Puzzle. Journal d'une Alzheimer* (Paris: Josette Lyon, 2004).
Crisp, Jane, Making sense of the stories that people with Alzheimer's tell: a journey with my mother, *Nursing Inquiry*, 2.3 (1995), 133–140.
'DASNI annual general meeting 17 April 2003 – minutes'; http://www.dasninternational.org/2003/2003agm_minutes.php (accessed August 2016).
Davidson, Ann, *Alzheimer's. A Love Story. One Year in My Husband's Journey* (Secaucus: Carol Publishing Group, 1997).
Davidson, Warren A. S., Metaphors of health and aging: geriatrics as metaphor, In *Metaphors of Aging in Science and the Humanities*, ed. by Gary M. Kenyon, James E. Birren and Johannes J. F. Schroots (New York: Springer Publishing Company, 1991), 173–198.
Davis, Boyd H., Introduction: some commonalities, In *Alzheimer Talk, Text and Context. Enhancing Communication*, ed. by Boyd H. Davis (New York: Palgrave Macmillan, 2008), xi–xxi.
Davis, Lennard J., *Enforcing Normalcy. Disability, Deafness, and the Body* (London: Verso, 1995).
Davis, Robert, *My Journey into Alzheimer's Disease. Helpful Insights for Family and Friends. A True Story* (Carol Stream: Tyndale House Publishers, 1989).
DeBaggio, Thomas, *Losing My Mind. An Intimate Look at Life with Alzheimer's* (New York: The Free Press, 2002).
DeBaggio, Thomas, *When it Gets Dark. An Enlightened Reflection on Life with Alzheimer's* (New York: The Free Press, 2003).
DeFalco, Amelia, *Uncanny Subjects. Aging in Contemporary Narrative* (Columbus: The Ohio State University Press, 2010).
DeFalco, Amelia, Dementia, caregiving, and narrative in Michael Ignatieff's *Scar Tissue, Occasion: Interdisciplinary Studies in the Humanities*, 4 (2012); http://arcade.stanford.edu/occasion/dementia-caregiving-and-narrative-michael-ignatieff%E2%80%99s-scar-tissue (accessed August 2016).
'Demenz Support Stuttgart. Philosophie'; http://www.demenz-support.de/portraet/philosophie (accessed August 2016).

Desai, Anita, The narrator has Alzheimer's, *New York Times*, 17 September 1989.
Diedrich, Lisa, *Treatments. Language, Politics, and the Culture of Illness* (Minneapolis: University of Minnesota Press, 2007).
Di Pietrantonio, Donatella, *Mia madre è un fiume* (Rome: Elliot Edizioni S. R. L., 2010).
Dolan, Josephine, Gordon, Suzy, and Estella Tincknell, The post-feminist biopic: re-telling the past in *Iris, The Hours* and *Sylvia*, In *Adaptation in Contemporary Culture. Textual Infidelities*, ed. by Rachel Carroll (London: Continuum, 2009), 174–185.
Donohue, Mike, *From AA to AD, a Wistful Travelogue* (Seattle: CreateSpace, 2009).
Eakin, Paul John, *How Our Lives Become Stories. Making Selves* (Ithaca: Cornell University Press, 1999).
Eakin, Paul John, *Living Autobiographically. How We Create Identity in Narrative* (Ithaca: Cornell University Press, 2008).
Edgar-Hunt, Robert, Marland, John, and Steven Rawle, *The Language of Film* (Lausanne: Ava Publishing S. A., 2010).
Egan, Timothy, 'Her mind was everything', dead woman's husband says, *New York Times*, 6 June 1990.
Ehrenreich, Barbara, *Smile or Die. How Positive Thinking Fooled America and the World* (London: Granta Books, 2010).
Elger, Katrin, Das Demenz-Dilemma, *Der Spiegel*, 19 September 2011.
Elliott, Anthony, *Concepts of the Self* (Cambridge: Polity Press, 2008).
Erlinger, Rainer, Vorgeführt im Verfall, *Süddeutsche Zeitung*, 5 February 2013.
Ernaux, Annie, *Une femme* (Paris: Éditions Gallimard, 1987); English version: *A Woman's Story*, trans. by Tanya Leslie (New York: Seven Stories Press, 1991).
Ernaux, Annie, *Je ne suis pas sortie de ma nuit* (Paris: Éditions Gallimard, 1997); English version: *I Remain in Darkness*, trans. by Tanya Leslie (New York: Seven Stories Press, 1999).
Espinel, Carlos H., de Kooning's late colours and forms: dementia, creativity, and the healing power of art, *The Lancet*, 347 (1996), 1096–1098.
Eyre, Richard, *Iris* (BBC, 2001).
Fine, Michelle, and Adrienne Asch, Introduction: beyond pedestals, In *Women with Disabilities: Essays in Psychology, Culture, and Politics*, ed. by Michelle Fine and Adrienne Asch (Philadelphia: Temple University Press, 1988), 1–37.
Finger, Stanley, The neuropathology of memory, In *Origins of Neuroscience* (New York: Oxford University Press, 1994), 349–368.
Fingerman, Karen L., Pitzer, Lindsay, Lefkowitz, Eva S., Birditt, Kira S., and Daniel Mroczek, Ambivalent relationship qualities between adults and their parents: implications for both parties' well-being, *The Journals of*

Gerontology, Series B: Psychological Sciences and Social Sciences, 63.6 (2008), P362–P371.

Floyd, Kory, and Mark T. Morman, Human affection exchange: affectionate communication in father–son relationships, *The Journal of Social Psychology*, 143.5 (2003), 599–612.

Fontana, Andrea, and Ronald W. Smith, Alzheimer's disease victims: the 'unbecoming' of self and the normalization of competence, *Sociological Perspectives*, 32 (1989), 35–46.

Fox, Judith, *I Still Do. Loving and Living with Alzheimer's* (New York: Power House Books, 2009).

Frank, Arthur W., *At the Will of the Body. Reflections on Illness* (Boston: Mariner Books, 2002).

Frank, Arthur W., *The Wounded Storyteller. Body, Illness, and Ethics* (Chicago: The University of Chicago Press, 1995).

Frank, Arthur W., Illness and autobiographical work: dialogue as narrative destabilization, *Qualitative Sociology*, 23.1 (2000), 135–156.

Franzen, Jonathan, My Father's Brain, In *How to Be Alone* (London: Fourth Estate, 2010), 7–38.

Fraser, Benjamin, *Disability Studies and Spanish Culture. Films, Novels, the Comic and the Public Exhibition* (Liverpool: Liverpool University Press, 2013).

Freadman, Richard, Decent and indecent: writing my father's life, In *The Ethics of Life Writing*, ed. by Paul John Eakin (Ithaca: Cornell University Press, 2004), 121–146.

Garrard, Peter, Maloney, Lisa M., Hodges, John R., and Karalyn Patterson, The effects of very early Alzheimer's disease on the characteristics of writing by a renowned author, *Brain*, 128 (2005), 250–260.

Geiger, Arno, *Der alte König in seinem Exil* (Munich: Carl Hanser, 2011).

Gentleman, Amelia, The raw horror of Alzheimer's, *The Guardian*, 1 June 2010.

Gillies, Andrea, *Keeper. Living with Nancy. A Journey into Alzheimer's* (London: Short Books, 2009).

Goyder, Julie, *We'll Be Married in Fremantle* (Fremantle: Fremantle Arts Centre Press, 2001).

Graboys, Thomas, with Peter Zheutlin, *Life in the Balance. A Physician's Memoir of Life, Love, and Loss with Parkinson's Disease and Dementia* (New York: Sterling Publishing, 2008).

Granser, Peter, *Alzheimer* (Heidelberg: Kehrer Verlag, 2008).

Grant, Linda, *Remind Me Who I Am, Again* (London: Granta Books, 1999).

Grant, Meg, Looking into her labyrinth, *People*, 22 March 1993.

Grothé, Jean, *Alzheimer. Un journal photographique* (Montreal: Les 400 coups, 2007).

Gubrium, Jaber, Narrative practice and the inner worlds of the Alzheimer disease experience, In *Concepts of Alzheimer Disease. Biological, Clinical, and Cultural*

Perspectives, ed. by Peter J. Whitehouse, Konrad Maurer and Jesse F. Ballenger (Baltimore: The Johns Hopkins University Press, 2000), 181–203.

Hadas, Rachel, *Strange Relation. A Memoir of Marriage, Dementia, and Poetry* (Philadelphia: Paul Dry Books, 2011).

Hadas, Rachel, Nothing's mortal enemy, *The Lancet*, 379 (2012), 2142–2143.

Hadler, Nortin M., *Rethinking Aging. Growing Old and Living Well in an Overtreated Society* (Chapel Hill: The University of North Carolina Press, 2011).

Hawkins, Anne Hunsaker, *Reconstructing Illness. Studies in Pathography*, 2nd edition (West Lafayette: Purdue University Press, 1999).

Hayes, Jeanne, Boylstein, Craig, and Mary K. Zimmerman, Living and loving with dementia: negotiating spousal and caregiver identity through narrative, *Journal of Aging Studies*, 23 (2009), 48–59.

'Helga Rohra – Im Dialog vom 17.02.2012'; http://www.youtube.com/watch?v=Bq6M_3uCqQQ (accessed August 2016).

Helmes, Edward, Merskey, Harold, Fox, Hannah, Fry, Richard N., Bowler, John V., and Vladimir C. Hachinski, Patterns of deterioration in senile dementia of the Alzheimer type, *Archives of Neurology*, 52.3 (1995), 306–310.

Henderson, Cary Smith, *Partial View. An Alzheimer's Journal* (Dallas: Southern Methodist University Press, 1998).

Herskovits, Elizabeth, Struggling over subjectivity: debates about the 'self' and Alzheimer's disease, *Medical Anthropology Quarterly*, 9.2 (1995), 146–164.

Hill, Robert, *Positive Aging. A Guide for Mental Health Professionals and Consumers* (New York: W. W. Norton, 2005).

Himmelfarb, Gertrude, A man's own household his enemies, *Commentary Magazine*, 108 (1999), 34–38.

Hinton, W. Ladson, and Sue Levkoff, Constructing Alzheimer's: narratives of lost identities, confusion and loneliness in old age, *Culture, Medicine and Psychiatry*, 23.4 (1999), 453–475.

'Hirnliga e. V. – Deutschlands Alzheimer Forscher'; http://www.hirnliga.de/index.html (accessed August 2016).

Hirst, Michael, Trends in informal care in Great Britain during the 1990s, *Health and Social Care in the Community*, 9.6 (2001), 348–357.

Holroyd, Michael, *Basil Street Blues. A Family Story* and *Mosaic* (London: Vintage, 2010).

Hughes, Julian C., Louw, Stephen J., and Steven R. Sabat, Seeing whole, In *Dementia. Mind, Meaning, and the Person*, ed. by Julian C. Hughes, Stephen J. Louw and Steven R. Sabat (New York: Oxford University Press, 2006), 1–39.

Hunter, Kathryn Montgomery, *Doctors' Stories. The Narrative Structure of Medical Knowledge* (Princeton: Princeton University Press, 1991).

Hydén, Lars-Christer, Narrative collaboration and scaffolding in dementia, *Journal of Aging Studies*, 25 (2011), 339–347.

Hydén, Lars-Christer, and L. Örulv, Narrative and identity in Alzheimer's disease: a case study, *Journal of Aging Studies*, 23 (2009), 205–214.
Ich bin dement, na und?, *Süddeutsche Zeitung*, 1 April 2010.
Ignatieff, Michael, *Scar Tissue* (London: Vintage, 1994).
Inoue, Yasushi, *Chronicle of My Mother*, trans. by Jean O. Moy (New York: Kodansha America, 1985).
'Im Fokus: Menschen mit Demenz – Wenn Praxis und Forschung verbunden werden'; http://www.nar.uni-heidelberg.de/veranstaltungen/kongress/archiv.html (accessed October 2016).
'*I Still Do* by Judith Fox'; https://www.youtube.com/watch?v=pWLhLD7Ox_g (accessed August 2016).
Jellinger, Kurt A., Neurobiology of cognitive impairment in Parkinson's disease, *Expert Review of Neurotherapeutics*, 12.12 (2012), 1451–1466.
Jens, Inge, *Unvollständige Erinnerungen* (Reinbeck bei Hamburg: Rowohlt, 2009).
Jens, Tilman, *Demenz. Abschied von meinem Vater* (Gütersloh: Gütersloher Verlagshaus, 2009).
Jens, Tilman, *Vatermord. Wider einen Generalverdacht* (Gütersloh: Gütersloher Verlagshaus, 2010).
Jens, Walter, and Hans Küng, *Menschenwürdig sterben. Ein Plädoyer für Selbstverantwortung* (Munich: Piper, 2009).
Jonsson, Carl-Otto, Edin, P., Söderberg, Siv, and Stig Waldton, Exploratory behavior in patients suffering from senile dementia: a comparison with children, *Acta Psychiatrica Scandinavica*, 53.4 (1976), 302–320.
Jurecic, Ann, *Illness as Narrative* (Pittsburgh: University of Pittsburgh Press, 2012).
Kitwood, Tom, The dialectics of dementia: with particular reference to Alzheimer's disease, *Ageing and Society*, 10 (1999), 177–196.
Kleinman, Arthur, *The Illness Narratives. Suffering, Healing, and the Human Condition* (New York: Basic Books, 1988).
Konek, Carol Wolfe, *Daddyboy. A Family's Struggle with Alzheimer's* (Saint Paul: Graywolf Press, 1991).
Kontos, Pia C., Embodied selfhood in Alzheimer's disease. Rethinking person-centred care, *Dementia*, 4 (2005), 553–570.
Kravitz, Bennett, *Representations of Illness in Literature and Film* (Newcastle upon Tyne: Cambridge Scholars Publishing, 2010).
Krémer, Pascale, Alzheimer. Récits d'un exil intérieur, *Le Monde 2*, 20 October 2007.
Laborde, Françoise, *Pourquoi ma mère me rend folle* (Paris: Flammarion, 2002).
Laborde, Françoise, *Ma mère n'est pas un philodendron* (Paris: Flammarion, 2003).
Lakoff, George, and Mark Johnson, *Metaphors We Live by* (Chicago: The University of Chicago Press, 2003).

Lanser, Susan S., Queering narratology, In *Ambiguous Discourse: Feminist Narratology and British Women Writers*, ed. by Kathy Mezei (Chapel Hill: The University of North Carolina Press, 1996), 250–261.
LaPlante, Alice, *Turn of Mind* (London: Harvill Secker, 2011).
Leavitt, Sarah, Kaddish, In *Beyond Forgetting. Poetry and Prose about Alzheimer's Disease*, ed. by Holly J. Hughes (Kent: The Kent State University Press, 2009), 167–168.
Leavitt, Sarah, *Tangles. A Story about Alzheimer's, My Mother, and Me* (London: Jonathan Cape, 2011).
Leder, Drew, *The Absent Body* (Chicago: The University of Chicago Press, 1990).
Lee, Jeanne L., *Just Love Me. My Life Turned Upside-Down by Alzheimer's* (West Lafayette: Purdue University Press, 2003).
Leibing, Annette, Divided gazes. Alzheimer's disease, the person within, and death in life, In *Thinking about Dementia: Culture, Loss, and the Anthropology of Senility*, ed. by Annette Leibing and Lawrence Cohen (New Brunswick: Rutgers University Press, 2006), 240–268.
Lewis, Roger, Oversexed, overpaid and underworked, *The Times*, 14 November 2015.
Lima, Julie C., Allen, Susan M., Goldschneider, Frances, and Orna Intrator, Spousal caregiving in late midlife versus older ages: implications of work and family obligations, *The Journals of Gerontology. Series B. Psychological Sciences and Social Sciences*, 63.4 (2008), S229–S238.
Lindbergh, Reeve, *No More Words. A Journal of My Mother, Anne Morrow Lindbergh* (New York: Touchstone, 2002).
Linke, Amina, Münchnerin (59): So lebe ich mit Demenz, *Münchner Abendzeitung*, 25 May 2012.
Linton, Simi, Reassigning meaning, In *The Disability Studies Reader, 3rd edition*, ed. by Lennard J. Davis (New York: Routledge, 2010), 223–236.
Luthmer-Lechner, Ulrike, Ich bin dement – na und?, *Göppinger Kreisnachrichten*, 14 March 2013.
Mace, Nancy L., and Peter V. Rabins, *The 36-Hour Day. A Family Guide to Caring for People Who Have Alzheimer Disease, Related Dementias, and Memory Loss, 5th edition* (Baltimore: The Johns Hopkins University Press, 2011).
Magnusson, Sally, *Where Memories Go. Why Dementia Changes Everything* (London: Two Roads, 2014).
Manning, Gerald F., Spinning the 'globe of memory': metaphor, literature, and aging, In *Metaphors of Aging in Science and the Humanities*, ed. by Gary M. Kenyon, James E. Birren and Johannes J. F. Schroots (New York: Springer Publishing Company, 1991), 37–55.
Mason, Mary G., The other voice: autobiographies of women writers, In *Autobiography. Essays Theoretical and Critical*, ed. by James Olney (Princeton: Princeton University Press, 1980), 207–235.

McDonagh, Patrick, *Idiocy. A Cultural History* (Liverpool: Liverpool University Press, 2008).
McGowin, Diana Friel, *Living in the Labyrinth. A Personal Journey through the Maze of Alzheimer's* (New York: Dell Publishing, 1993).
McLean, Athena Helen, Coherence without facticity in dementia: the case of Mrs. Fine, In *Thinking about Dementia: Culture, Loss, and the Anthropology of Senility*, ed. by Annette Leibing and Lawrence Cohen (New Brunswick: Rutgers University Press, 2006), 157–179.
Merlin, Helen, Ich will integriert werden!, In *'Ich spreche für mich selbst.' Menschen mit Demenz melden sich zu Wort*, ed. by Demenz Support Stuttgart (Frankfurt am Main: Mabuse-Verlag, 2010), 11–24.
Michel, Bettina, with Eva Mohr, *Papa, ich bin für Dich da. Wie Sie Demenzkranken helfen können* (Munich: mvg Verlag, 2014).
Miller, Bruce L., Cummings, Jeffrey L., Mishkin, Fred, Boone, Kyle, Prince, François, Ponton, Michel, and Carl Cotman, Emergence of artistic talent in frontotemporal dementia, *Neurology*, 51 (1998), 978–981.
Mills, Claudia, Friendship, fiction, and memoir: trust and betrayal in writing from one's own life, In *The Ethics of Life Writing*, ed. by Paul John Eakin (Ithaca: Cornell University Press, 2004), 101–120.
Mintz, Susannah B., *Unruly Bodies. Life Writing by Women with Disabilities* (Chapel Hill: The University of North Carolina Press, 2007).
Mobley, Tracy, *Young Hope. The Broken Road* (Denver: Outskirts Press, 2007).
Morrison, John H., and Patrick R. Hof, Selective vulnerability of corticocortical and hippocampal circuits in aging and Alzheimer's disease, *Progress in Brain Research*, 136 (2002), 467–486.
'Mr Toledano. *Days with My Father*'; http://www.mrtoledano.com/days-with-my-father/01-Days-with-my-father (accessed August 2016).
Müller, Nicole, and Robert W. Schrauf, Conversation as cognition. Reframing cognition in dementia, In *Dialogue and Dementia. Cognitive and Communicative Resources for Engagement*, ed. by Robert W. Schrauf and Nicole Müller (New York: Psychology Press, 2014), 3–26.
Naue, Ursula, and Thilo Kroll, 'The demented other': identity and difference in dementia, *Nursing Philosophy*, 10 (2009), 26–33.
Navon, Liora, and Nurit Weinblatt, 'The show must go on': behind the scenes of elderly spousal caregiving, *Journal of Aging Studies*, 10.4 (1996), 329–342.
Neuman, Shirley, Autobiography and questions of gender: an introduction, *Prose Studies*, 14.2 (1991), 1–11.
Nüchterlein, Birgit, Zuhause ist jetzt anderswo, *Nürnberger Nachrichten*, 16 February 2011.
O'Rourke, Norm, Alzheimer's disease as a metaphor for contemporary fears of aging, *Journal of the American Geriatrics Society*, 44 (1996), 220–221.

Olney, James, *Metaphors of Self. The Meaning of Autobiography* (Princeton: Princeton University Press, 1972).
Orr, David M. R., and Yugin Teo, Carers' responses to shifting identity in dementia in *Iris* and *Away From Her*: cultivating stability or embracing change?, *Medical Humanities*, 41 (2015), 81–85.
Pachana, Nancy A., Boone, Kyle B., Miller, Bruce L., Cummings, Jeffrey L., and Nancy Berman, Comparison of neuropsychological functioning in Alzheimer's disease and frontotemporal dementia, *Journal of the International Neuropsychological Society*, 2 (1996), 505–510.
Papagno, Costanza, Comprehension of metaphors and idioms in patients with Alzheimer's disease, *Brain*, 124 (2001), 1450–1460.
Pease, Allan, and Barbara Pease, *The Definitive Book of Body Language* (London: Orion, 2005).
Perry, John, Diminished and fractured selves, In *Personal Identity and Fractured Selves*, ed. by Debra J. H. Mathews, Hilary Bok and Peter V. Rabins (Baltimore: The Johns Hopkins University Press, 2009), 129–162.
Pezzini, Liliana E., Pollak, Robert A., and Barbara S. Schone, Long-term care of the disabled elderly: do children increase caregiving by spouses?, *Review of Economics of the Household*, 7.3 (2009), 323–339.
Pierce, Charles P., *Hard to Forget. An Alzheimer's Story* (New York: Random House, 2000).
'Potsdamer Filmgespräch. *Vergiss Mein Nicht*'; http://www.kreatives-branden burg.de/veranstaltung/potsdamer-filmgesprach-vergiss-mein-nicht/ (accessed August 2016).
Pöysti, Minna M., Laakkonen, Marja-Liisa, Strandberg, Timo, Savikko, Niina, Tilvis, Reijo S., Eloniemi-Sulkava, Ulla, and Kaisu H. Pitkälä, Gender differences in dementia spousal caregiving, *International Journal of Alzheimer's Disease*, article 162960 (2012).
Price, Elizabeth, Coming out to care: gay and lesbian carers' experiences of dementia services, *Health and Social Care in the Community*, 18 (2010), 160–168.
Radisch, Iris, Der Mann seines Lebens. Tilman Jens verklärt und denunziert seinen an Demenz erkrankten wehrlosen Vater Walter Jens, *Die Zeit*, 19 February 2009.
Radley, Alan, *Works of Illness. Narrative, Picturing and the Social Response to Serious Disease* (Ashby-de-la-Zouch: Inkermen Press, 2009).
Ramanathan, Vai, *Alzheimer Discourse. Some Sociolinguistic Dimensions* (Mahwah: Lawrence Erlbaum Associates, 1997).
Ramanathan, Vaidehi, Alzheimer pathographies. Glimpses into how people with AD and their caregivers text themselves, In *Dialogue and Dementia. Cognitive and Communicative Resources for Engagement*, ed. by Robert W. Schrauf and Nicole Müller (New York: Psychology Press, 2014), 245–261.

Ray, Ruth E., The uninvited guest: mother/daughter conflict in feminist gerontology, *Journal of Aging Studies*, 17 (2003), 113–128.
'Reading guide. *Tangles*. Sarah Leavitt'; http://www.freehand-books.com/wp-content/uploads/2012/03/Tangles-Reading-Guide.pdf (accessed December 2016).
Ribeiro, Oscar, Paúl, Constança, and Conceição Nogueira, Real men, real husbands: caregiving and masculinities in later life, *Journal of Aging Studies*, 21 (2007), 302–313.
Riley II, Charles A., *Disability & the Media. Prescriptions for Change* (Lebanon: University Press of New England, 2005).
Rimmon-Kenan, Shlomith, The story of 'I': illness and narrative identity, *Narrative*, 10.1 (2002), 9–27.
Roach, Marion, Another name for madness, *New York Times Magazine*, 16 January 1983.
Rohra, Helga, *Aus dem Schatten treten. Warum ich mich für unsere Rechte als Demenzbetroffene einsetze* (Frankfurt am Main: Mabuse-Verlag, 2011).
Rose, Irene, Autistic autobiography or autistic life narrative?, *Journal of Literary Disability*, 2.1 (2008), 44–54.
Rose, Larry, *Show Me the Way to Go Home* (Forest Knolls: Elder Books, 1996).
Rose, Larry, *Larry's Way. Another Look at Alzheimer's from the Inside* (Lincoln: iUniverse, 2003).
Rota, Nucci A., *La bimbamamma. Cosa vuol dire convivere con l'Alzheimer. Il diario di una figlia* (Naples: Iuppiter Edizioni, 2009).
Rowe, Anne, Critical reception in England of *Iris: A Memoir of Iris Murdoch* by John Bayley, *Iris Murdoch Newsletter*, 13 (1999), 9–10.
Ryan, Ellen Bouchard, Bannister, Karen A., and Ann P. Anas, The dementia narrative: writing to reclaim social identity, *Journal of Aging Studies*, 23 (2009), 145–157.
Sabat, Steven R., *The Experience of Alzheimer's Disease. Life through a Tangled Veil* (Oxford: Blackwell Publishers Ltd., 2001).
Scarry, Elaine, *The Body in Pain. The Making and Unmaking of the World* (New York: Oxford University Press, 1985).
Schechtman, Marya, Getting our stories straight. Self-narrative and personal identity, In *Personal Identity and Fractured Selves*, ed. by Debra J. H. Mathews, Hilary Bok and Peter V. Rabins (Baltimore: The Johns Hopkins University Press, 2009), 65–92.
Schneider, Charles, *Don't Bury Me, It Ain't Over Yet!* (Bloomington: Author House, 2006).
Segers, Kurt, Degenerative dementias and their medical care in the movies, *Alzheimer Disease and Associated Disorders*, 21 (2007), 55–59.
Shenk, David, *The Forgetting. Alzheimer's: Portrait of an Epidemic* (New York: Anchor Books, 2003).

Shenk, Dena, There was an old woman: maintenance of identity by people with Alzheimer's dementia, In *Alzheimer Talk, Text and Context. Enhancing Communication*, ed. by Boyd H. Davis (New York: Palgrave Macmillan, 2008), 3–17.

Siegler, Ilene C., Brummett, Beverly H., Williams, Redford B., Haney, Thomas L., and Peggye Dilworth-Anderson, Caregiving, residence, race, and depressive symptoms, *Aging & Mental Health*, 14.7 (2010), 771–778.

Sieveking, David, *Vergiss Mein Nicht. Wie meine Mutter ihr Gedächtnis verlor und meine Eltern die Liebe neu entdeckten* (Farbfilm Verleih, 2012).

Sieveking, David, *Vergiss Mein Nicht. Wie meine Mutter ihr Gedächtnis verlor und ich meine Eltern neu entdeckte* (Freiburg im Breisgau: Herder, 2013).

Smith, James A., Braunack-Mayer, Annette, Wittert, Gary, and Megan Warin, 'I've been independent for so damn long!': independence, masculinity and aging in a help seeking context, *Journal of Aging Studies*, 21 (2007), 325–335.

Smith, Sidonie, and Julia Watson, *Reading Autobiography. A Guide for Interpreting Life Narratives* (Minneapolis: University of Minnesota Press, 2001).

Snyder, Lisa, *Speaking Our Minds. What It's Like to Have Alzheimer's* (Baltimore: Health Professions Press, 2009).

Sontag, Susan, *Illness as Metaphor* and *AIDS and Its Metaphors* (London: Penguin, 2002).

Sontag, Susan, *Regarding the Pain of Others* (London: Penguin, 2004).

Spohr, Betty Baker, with Jean Valens Bullard, *Catch a Falling Star. Living with Alzheimer's* (Seattle: Storm Peak Press, 1995).

Squiers, Carol, Ed Kashi. Aging in America, In *The Body at Risk. Photography of Disorder, Illness, and Healing* (Berkeley: University of California Press, 2005), 192–209.

Stanley, Patricia Haas, The patient's voice: a cry in solitude or a call for community, *Literature and Medicine*, 23.2 (2004), 346–363.

Strawson, Galen, Telling tales, *The Guardian*, 6 September 2003.

Stuckey, Jon C., Blessed assurance. The role of religion and spirituality in Alzheimer's disease caregiving and other significant life events, *Journal of Aging Studies*, 15 (2001), 69–84.

Tan, Tracy, and Margaret A. Schneider, Humor as a coping strategy for adult-child caregivers of individuals with Alzheimer's disease, *Geriatric Nursing*, 30 (2009), 397–408.

Taylor, Janelle S., On recognition, caring, and dementia, *Medical Anthropology Quarterly*, 22.4 (2008), 313–335.

Taylor, Richard, *Alzheimer's from the Inside Out* (Baltimore: Health Professions Press, 2007).

'The Trebus Project'; http://www.trebusprojects.org/ (accessed October 2016).

Toledano, Phillip, *Days with My Father* (San Francisco: Chronicle Books, 2010).

Traphagan, John W., Being a good *rōjin*: senility, power, and self-actualization in Japan, In *Thinking about Dementia: Culture, Loss, and the Anthropology of Senility*, ed. by Annette Leibing and Lawrence Cohen (New Brunswick: Rutgers University Press, 2006), 269–287.

Ueding, Gert, Tilman Jens begräbt den lebendigen Vater, *Die Welt*, 18 February 2009.

Van Vliet, Deliane, de Vugt, Marjolein E., Bakker, Christian, Koopmans, Raymond T. C. M, and Frans R. J. Verhey, Impact of early onset dementia on caregivers: a review, *International Journal of Geriatric Psychiatry*, 25.11 (2010), 1091–1100.

Venturino, Giovanna, *Il tuo mare di nulla. La mia mamma e l'Alzheimer* (Rome: A&B Editrice, 2012).

Vickers, Neil, Illness narratives, In *A History of English Autobiography*, ed. by Adam Smyth (New York: Cambridge University Press, 2016), 388–401.

Vingerhoets, Ad J. J. M., and Guus L. van Heck, Gender, coping and psychosomatic symptoms, *Psychological Medicine*, 20.1 (1990), 125–135.

Waddell, Margot, Only connect: developmental issues from early to late life, *Psychoanalytic Psychotherapy*, 14 (2000), 239–252.

Wall, Frank, *Where Did Mary Go? A Loving Husband's Struggle with Alzheimer's* (Amherst: Prometheus Books, 1996).

Westmacott, Robyn, Black, Sandra E., Freedman, Morris, and Morris Moscovitch, The contribution of autobiographical significance to semantic memory: evidence from Alzheimer's disease, semantic dementia, and amnesia, *Neuropsychologia*, 42.1 (2004), 25–48.

Whitehouse, Peter J., Losing my mind. An intimate look at life with Alzheimer's, *New England Journal of Medicine*, 347.11 (2002), 861.

Wilhoit, Mary, *As She Was Dying. An Alzheimer's Journal* (Lincoln: iUniverse, 2008).

Wilkinson, Jane, Remembering forgetting, *Status Quaestionis*, 6 (2014), 103–121.

Williams, Ian, Graphic medicine: how comics are revolutionizing the representation of illness, *Hektoen International. A Journal of Medical Humanities*, 3 (2012); http://www.hektoeninternational.org/index.php?option=com_content&view=article&id=353:graphic-medicine&catid=93&Itemid=716 (accessed August 2016).

Wilson, A. N., *Iris Murdoch as I Knew Her* (London: Arrow Books, 2004).

Wiltshire, John, Biography, pathography, and the recovery of meaning, *The Cambridge Quarterly*, 29 (2000), 409–422.

Wolk, Douglas, *Reading Comics. How Graphic Novels Work and What They Mean* (Cambridge: Da Capo Press, 2007).

Woodward, Kathleen, Reminiscence and the life review: prospects and retrospects, In *What Does It Mean to Grow Old? Reflections from the Humanities*, ed. by Thomas R. Cole and Sally Gadow (Durham: Duke University Press, 1986), 135–161.

Yahnke, Robert E., Old age and loss in feature-length films, *The Gerontologist*, 43 (2003), 426–428.
Yahnke, Robert E., and Richard M. Eastman, *Literature and Gerontology. A Research Guide* (Westport: Greenwood Press, 1995).
Zabbia, Kim Howes, *Painted Diaries. A Mother and Daughter's Experience through Alzheimer's* (Minneapolis: Fairview Press, 1996).
Zacharias, Sylvia, *Diagnose Alzheimer: Helmut Zacharias. Ein Bericht* (Cologne: Hirnliga e. V., 2000).
Zeilig, Hannah, The critical use of narrative and literature in gerontology, *International Journal of Ageing and Later Life*, 6.2 (2011), 7–37.
Zeilig, Hannah, Dementia as a cultural metaphor, *The Gerontologist*, 54 (2014), 258–267.
Zimmermann, Christian, and Peter Wißmann, *Auf dem Weg mit Alzheimer. Wie sich mit einer Demenz leben lässt* (Frankfurt am Main: Mabuse-Verlag, 2011).
Zimmermann, Martina, Deliver us from evil: carer burden in Alzheimer's disease, *Medical Humanities*, 36 (2010), 101–107.
Zimmermann, Martina, Dementia in life-writing: our health care system in the words of the sufferer, *Neurological Sciences*, 32 (2011), 1233–1238.
Zimmermann, Martina, Narrating stroke: the life-writing and fiction of brain damage, *Medical Humanities*, 38 (2012), 73–77.
Zimmermann, Martina, Integrating medical humanities into a pharmaceutical care seminar on dementia, *American Journal of Pharmaceutical Education*, 77.1 (2013a), article 16.
Zimmermann, Martina, 'Journeys' in the life-writing of adult-child dementia caregivers, *Journal of Medical Humanities*, 34 (2013b), 385–397.
Zimmermann, Martina, Alzheimer's disease metaphors as mirror and lens to the stigma of dementia, *Literature and Medicine* (forthcoming Spring 2017).

Index

A
Acceptance, 27, 77, 80, 100, 107, 108
Account
   chronological, 113, 130
   co-authored, collaborative, 21, 86, 99
   fragmented, 28, 78, 83, 84, 89, 90, 96, 105, 107, 108
   linear, 21, 78, 96
   seamless, 94
   snippets, 31, 64, 66
   See also Diary; Essay; Graphic novel; Journal; Pathography; Photo; Picture book
Active, 20, 22, 27, 31, 39, 42, 43, 45, 61, 63, 101, 102, 106
Activism, 21, 91, 97, 98–103, 116
Advanced directive, 93
   See also Assisted suicide; Euthanasia
Advocacy, 1–22, 77, 80
Agency, 57, 60, 72, 86, 88, 100, 106, 107, 109, 120, 128
Aging, 3, 14, 20, 21, 28, 50–73, 91, 100, 103, 119, 128–132
Allegory, Alzheimer's disease as, 3, 50, 66, 90–91
   See also Postmodern

Alzheimer's Disease International (ADI), 4, 102
Alzheimer's disease
   diagnosis, 2, 3, 9, 33, 34, 39, 83, 86–88, 93, 99, 100, 103, 104, 106, 109, 112, 113, 120, 125
   epidemiology, prevalence, incidence, 3, 15, 96, 110
   stages, 69, 86
   See also Dementia
Alzheimer's from the Inside Out, 101–103
   See also Taylor, Richard
Ambivalence, 59, 72, 109
America, American, 3, 7, 15, 50, 52, 53, 63, 76
Anger, 34, 92–93, 101
Appignanesi, Josh, 52, 70–72, 77
Aronson, Jeffrey, 6
Artist, artistic, 11, 16, 26, 89, 90, 94, 107, 109
Asia, 131
   See also China; India
Asperger's syndrome, 112
   See also Autism
Assauer, Rudi, 114–115

INDEX

Assisted suicide, 57
　See also Advanced directive; End-of-life; Euthanasia
Attention span, 21, 83, 84, 98, 101
Audience, 5, 16, 77–78, 97, 125, 127
Aus dem Schatten treten, 110–116
　See also Rohra, Helga
Australia, Australian, 4, 15
Austria, Austrian, 4, 52, 65, 68
Authority, 12, 17, 34, 90, 91–94, 95–116
Autism, 90, 122
　See also Asperger's syndrome
Autonomy, 21, 64, 67, 69, 108, 110, 118
A Woman's Story, 29
　See also Ernaux, Annie

B

Ballenger, Jesse F., 85, 89, 106
Basting, Anne Davis, 2, 7, 11, 20, 81, 84, 102
Battle, *see* Images
Bayley, John, 5, 6, 24–25, 51–57, 60, 61, 68, 90, 126–127
Beast, *see* Images
Behaviour, 25, 30, 40–44, 56, 60, 71, 73, 102
Biomedical, 4, 11, 18, 119
Biopsychosocial, 41
Black, blackness, *see* Images
Blank, blankness, *see* Images
Blog, 16, 28, 64
　See also Online
Blurred, faded, 36, 59, 63, 106
Boat, *see* Images
Boden, Christine, 76, 77, 103
　See also Bryden, Christine
Bodily, 11, 37, 57, 60, 68, 86, 97
Body, 7, 52–62, 76, 90, 93, 97, 103, 119

Book
　book-length, 5, 8, 76, 128
　market, 16, 128
　print-on-demand, 16, 17, 20, 101
Bradford Dementia Group, 71
Bright, brightness, *see* Images
Britain, British, 7, 51, 53, 55, 96
　See also England, English; United Kingdom
Brockmeier, Jens, 61, 131
Brody, Howard, 8
Bruner, Jerome, 9
Bryden, Christine, 97, 103–107, 109, 112, 116, 118
　See also Boden, Christine
Buades, Margarita Retuerto, 24, 42, 51
Burack-Weiss, Ann, 19
Burden, caregiver duty, 4, 15, 16, 19, 20, 27, 32, 35, 40–46, 51, 69, 76, 115, 119, 121, 128, 132
Burke, Lucy, 11, 28, 85, 119
Bury, Michael, 31

C

Canada, Canadian, 4, 52, 58
Candor, 51, 101
Care, caregiving
　burden, 4, 19, 27, 32, 40–46, 51, 119, 132 (*see also* Stress)
　caregiver-centred, 20, 26, 110
　drain, exhaustion, 65, 119, 127
　duty, 19
　hands-on, 20, 25, 27, 38;
　　bathing, clothing, 45, 71, 121, 122;
　　feeding, 34, 45, 122
　patient-centred, 20, 22, 27, 77, 82, 101, 102, 110
　person-centred, 72
Career, 33, 79, 92, 114, 126

Caregiver, carer
  familial, 17, 51
  guide, *see* Manual
  professional, 17, 25, 34, 51, 54, 92
Catch a Falling Star, 33–35
  See also Spohr, Betty Baker
Chaos narrative, 8, 25, 84, 85, 103
  See also Frank, Arthur W.
Charon, Rita, 63, 129
Child
  adult child, 18, 19, 26, 27–33, 40, 41, 44, 51, 52, 65, 69, 100, 115, 118, 119
  parent turned child, 41, 46, 51
Childhood, return to, second, 30, 40, 60, 102
Childlike, 30, 40, 44, 60, 61
China, 131
  See also Asia
Chivers, Sally, 15
Chronic, chronicity, 4, 7, 17–18, 79, 80, 91, 103
Chronicle, 27, 58, 63, 105
  See also Account – chronological, linear, seamless
Clinician, 78, 131
  See also Doctor; Physician
Closeness, close contact, 53, 55
Cognition
  cognitive challenge, 73, 82, 101, 105, 108
  cognitive impairment, 7, 9, 13, 21, 69, 96, 115
Cohen, Lawrence, 76, 77, 87, 93, 131
Coherence, *vs.* jumbled, 8–10, 67, 83, 97, 120, 129
Colour, 106, 108, 109
Comic, *see* Graphic novel
Companionship, 38, 42, 53, 110
Contents, *vs.* form, 21, 83–91, 99, 106, 123
Continuity, creation of, 27, 28, 31–33, 41, 51, 53, 56, 67, 80, 81, 101, 129

Control, 35, 39, 128
Conway, Kathlyn, 7, 8, 85, 91–93
Coping
  detachment, impersonal, 29, 34–35, 51, 59, 107
  devises, strategies, 14, 25, 35, 41, 70, 105, 107, 109
Corporeal, 50
Couple, 26, 36, 37, 43, 53, 54, 57
  See also Husband; Partner; Spouse; Wife
Couser, G. Thomas, 13, 15, 20, 22, 62, 78, 128
Couturier, Claude, 97, 107–109, 112, 116
Cover, book, DVD, 32, 43, 101, 106, 111, 124, 125
Creativity, 26, 33, 38, 107–109
Crisis, 11, 52, 104, 130

D

Daddyboy, 30–33
  See also Konek, Carol Wolfe
Dance, *see* Images
Dancing with Dementia, 103–107
  See also Bryden, Christine
Darkness, dark, *see* Images
Daughter, 23–46, 50, 63, 68, 70, 84, 85, 109, 119, 121–123
Davidson, Ann, 34
Davis, Lennard J., 97
Davis, Robert, 5, 11, 78–83, 91, 100, 103–106, 108, 109
Days with My Father, 62–65
  See also Toledano, Phillip
Death, dying, 3, 4, 18, 27–29, 31–33, 35, 41, 50, 54, 55, 63, 64, 67, 80, 82, 86–89, 92, 93, 101, 107, 108, 120, 126, 129, 130
Death sentence, *see* Images

DeBaggio, Thomas, 78, 86–91, 97, 100, 104, 106–108, 112, 125, 131
Decision, end-of-life, 32, 78, 99, 125, 126
DeFalco, Amelia, 24, 54
Degeneration, 4, 7, 13, 18, 66, 79, 91, 103, 108
Dementia
  early-onset, 3, 113, 115
  early-stage, 3, 107, 115, 128, 132
  late-onset, 3
  late-stage, 3, 69, 115, 128
  See also Frontotemporal dementia; Lewy body dementia; Parkinson's disease
Dementia Advocacy and Support Network International (DASNI), 80–81, 98, 102, 105
Denial, 7, 81
Dependence, 4, 21, 52, 53, 54, 62, 81, 98, 109, 119, 129
  See also Independence
Der alte König in seinem Exil, 65–68, 118
  See also Geiger, Arno
Description, *vs.* performance of disease, 3, 11, 21, 42, 46, 68, 83–85, 88, 89, 106
Despair, 36, 57, 79, 91, 92, 120
Detachment, 29, 34–35, 51, 107
  See also Coping
Diary, 27–30, 53, 64, 97–98, 107–108, 120, 122, 124
  See also Account; Essay; Graphic novel; Journal
Diedrich, Lisa, 54, 56
Dignity, 13, 63, 86, 126
Di Pietrantonio, Donatella, 118
Disability, 7, 14–15, 18, 96–97
Disorientation, 36, 66, 86
Disruption, biographical, 9, 12, 24, 31, 67, 70, 77, 79, 90, 91, 97

See also Bury, Michael
Doctor, 33–34, 92–93, 99, 100, 108, 113, 121
  See also Clinician; Physician
Documentary, 119, 125
Dog, *see* Images
Donohue, Mike, 103, 106
Drawing
  cartoon, caricature, 26, 33–35, 119–123
  expressionistic *vs.* impressionistic, 109
  See also Painting; Picture book
Drugs, 3, 18, 84, 91, 99
Dysnarrativia, 9, 13

E

Eakin, Paul John, 8–9, 54, 82–83
Education, 19, 51, 68, 132
  See also Upbringing
Elderly, 2, 3, 5, 19, 59, 62, 89, 113, 115, 131
Eloquence, 82, 88, 98
Embodiment, 60–61
Empathy, 43, 61, 62, 122
Emptiness, 60, 120
End-of-life, 8, 32, 78, 99, 125, 126
England, English, 15, 27, 29, 38
  See also Britain, British; United Kingdom
Ernaux, Annie, 26–32, 34, 39–42, 44, 63, 65–67, 69, 84, 105, 108, 119, 121
Essay, 68, 90, 98, 101, 105, 106
  See also Diary; Journal
Ethicality, 42, 63
  Ethical implications, 7, 13, 56
Ethnicity, 19
Europe, European, 4, 15, 57, 76, 85
Euthanasia, 76
  See also Advanced directive; Assisted suicide

Exile, *see* Images
Ex Memoria, 52, 69–72
 See also Appignanesi, Josh
Eye contact, 59, 60, 70, 72, 85, 111
 See also Gaze
Eyre, Richard, 5, 54, 61

F
Faith, 80, 81, 103, 104, 109
 See also God; Religion; Spirituality
Famous, celebrity patient, 57
 See also Prominent
Fear, of diagnosis, of loss, 3, 4, 6, 12, 31, 46, 50, 66, 87, 92, 97, 102, 119, 128, 130
Film, 16, 51, 52, 54, 60, 70–73, 123–127
 See also Appignanesi, Josh; Eyre, Richard; Sieveking, David
Forgetfulness, 99
Form, *vs.* contents, 3, 11, 21, 26, 29, 31, 83–91, 97, 99, 101, 106, 121, 123, 130
Foucault, Michel, 83
Fox, Judith, 26, 36–38, 41, 42, 45, 61–64, 85, 118, 121
France, French, 4, 15, 28–29, 63
Frank, Arthur W., 8, 14, 17, 25, 56, 79, 84, 91
Franzen, Jonathan, 90
Freedom, 21, 34, 42, 72, 102, 121
Friends, 40, 43, 92, 99, 112, 116, 123
Frontotemporal dementia, 18, 104, 106
 See also Dementia
Frustration, 93, 113, 123, 129
Fun, 42, 63, 107
 See also Humour; Irony; Laughter
Future, *see* Past

G
Gaze, 59, 62, 63, 71, 72, 86
 See also Eye contact

Geiger, Arno, 52, 62, 65–69, 79, 89–90, 100, 118, 124, 126, 130
Gender, 14, 19–21, 45, 51, 52, 68, 94, 97, 109
Generational, 19, 33
German, Germany, 4, 15, 52, 55, 58, 71, 110–111, 114, 118–119, 125
Gillies, Andrea, 24, 33, 51, 57, 65, 67
God, 107
 See also Faith; Religion; Spirituality
Graboys, Thomas, 78, 92–94, 99, 102, 125
Grant, Linda, 31
Graphic novel, 16
 See also Account; Diary; Essay; Journal
Gratitude, 24, 105
Grief, hardship, 4, 129
Grothé, Jean, 52, 58–61, 63, 64, 68, 79, 86, 100, 111, 127
Growth, 26, 32, 104–105
Guilt, 34, 129

H
Hadas, Rachel, 26, 38–43, 53, 118, 129
Happiness, happy, 44, 53, 101, 127
Hawkins, Anne Hunsaker, 13, 22, 28, 66, 78, 79, 81, 104
 See also Images; Myth
Healing, 29, 77, 79, 132
Henderson, Cary Smith, 11, 78, 83–86, 89–91, 97, 99, 106, 108, 111
Heterosexist, 122
Holocaust of the brain, *see* Images
Holroyd, Michael, 50, 55
Home
 care home, nursing home, 27, 32, 33, 38, 39, 59, 64, 69–72
 household help, 38
 institution, institutionalisation, 39, 96
 placement, 129

Honesty, 72, 98, 116, 119, 121
Hospital, 17, 59, 125–126
Humour, 42, 44–45, 101, 107
   See also Fun; Irony; Laughter
Hunter, Kathryn Montgomery, 34
Husband, 13, 20, 25, 26, 33–39, 41, 45, 53, 57, 60, 62, 64, 83, 84, 86, 126, 129
   See also Couple; Partner; Spouse

I

Identity
   affirming, 14, 51, 62, 129
   denying, 12, 52, 61
   patient, post-autobiographical, pre-narrative, 7–22, 60–63
Ignatieff, Michael, 24–25, 50
Images
   battle, 107, 113
   beast, 81
   blackness, black, 112, 120, 123, 127
   blankness, blank, 63
   boat, 53
   brightness, bright, 79, 89, 106, 109, 120
   dance, 106
   darkness, dark, 37, 53, 79–80, 108, 111, 112, 120, 126
   death sentence, 86, 107
   dog, 35
   exile, 66
   holocaust of the brain, 86–87
   intruder, 81
   journey, 13, 37, 62, 78–83, 99, 100, 104, 106, 109, 127, 129
   killer, 84
   labyrinth, maze, 5, 83
   maimer, 84
   pearl, 111
   phoenix, 104, 112
   rebirth, 104
   river, 53, 64, 109, 118
   shadow, 36, 43, 63, 83, 92, 111, 112, 120, 125
   shell, 104–105
   ship, 59
   torture, 87
   vegetable, 107
   verdict, 32, 33, 80
   victim, 2, 76, 78, 80–81, 87, 93, 109, 126
Independence, 21, 57, 63, 86, 101, 109, 115, 129
   See also Dependence
India, 15, 76, 131
   See also Asia
Infantilising, 67, 73, 102, 131
Institution, institutionalisation, see Home
Intellectual, 3, 14, 38, 42, 52, 57, 61, 80, 96, 101
Interview, 16, 17, 111, 114, 121
Intruder, see Images
I Remain in Darkness, 27–28
   See also Ernaux, Annie
Iris: A Memoir, 51, 53–57, 90
   See also Bayley, John
Irony, 72, 101
   See also Fun; Humour; Laughter
I Still Do, 36–38
   See also Fox, Judith
Italian, Italy, 4, 15, 29, 52, 63

J

Japan, Japanese, 15, 50, 68
Jens, Inge, 57, 93
Jens, Tilman, 52, 55–58, 60, 61, 64, 68, 85, 101, 115
Jens, Walter, 57, 69, 81, 93, 107, 126
Johnson, Mark, 35, 79
Journal, 50, 59, 83, 84, 86, 99, 108
   See also Account; Diary; Essay; Graphic novel

Journey, *see* Images
Joy, *see* Happiness
Jurecic, Ann, 14
Just Love Me, 98–100
    See also Lee, Jeanne L.

K
Kevorkian, Jack, 76
Killer, *see* Images
Kitwood, Tom, 66
Kleinman, Arthur, 35
Konek, Carol Wolfe, 26, 30–33, 37, 40, 43, 64, 65, 67, 69, 79, 89, 121, 124
Kontos, Pia C., 61
Kübler-Ross, Elisabeth, 82

L
Laborde, Françoise, 28
Labyrinth, *see* Images
Lakoff, George, 35, 79
Larry's Way, 81, 83
    See also Rose, Larry
Laughter, 2
    See also Fun; Humour; Irony
Leavitt, Sarah, 119–123
Lee, Jeanne L., 97–100, 102, 105, 113
Legacy, 57, 88
Lesbian, 122
Lewy body dementia, 18, 78, 92, 110
    See also Dementia
Life in the Balance, 92–94
    See also Graboys, Thomas
Lindbergh, Reeve, 27, 42–46, 67–69, 102, 124, 129
Linguistic, 7, 9, 88, 102, 105, 126
Living in the Labyrinth, 5, 79, 81–82
    See also McGowin, Diana Friel
Loneliness, lonely, 38–40, 87, 120, 121

Losing My Mind, 86–88
    See also DeBaggio, Thomas
Loss, *see* Fear; Memory

M
Mace, Nancy L., 34
Magnusson, Sally, 118
Maimer, *see* Images
Manual, caregiver guide, 34, 35
Marriage, 35, 37, 39, 53, 57, 92, 99, 127
Maze, *see* Images – labyrinth
McGowin, Diana Friel, 5, 11, 78, 81–83, 91, 100, 102, 105, 106, 109, 112
Medico-scientific
    discourse, 2, 18, 22, 32, 77
    research, 3, 4, 127
Memoir, *see* Account; Diary; Essay; Graphic novel; Journal
Memory
    erosion, 4, 82, 124
    long-term *vs.* short-term, 87
    loss, 3–7, 25, 44, 57, 65, 73, 80, 82, 89, 90, 106, 107, 129
Metaphors, 30, 33–34, 36, 44, 51, 55, 60, 72, 79–81, 83, 86–88, 104–108, 112, 121, 130
    See also Images
Midlife, 38, 115
Mind-defined, 57, 102
    See also Intellectual
Mobley, Tracy, 81, 96, 113
Modern, *vs.* postmodern, 89–90
Movie, *see* Film
Murdoch, Iris, 51, 53–56, 61, 69, 90, 126–127
My Journey into Alzheimer's Disease, 5, 78–81
    See also Davis, Robert
Myth, 13, 14, 22, 78, 79, 104

Myth (*cont.*)
  formulation, 13, 79, 129
  See also Images; Hawkins, Anne Hunsaker

N

No More Words, 42–45
  See also Lindbergh, Reeve
Norms, 9, 17, 91–94, 96–97, 115
Nursing home, *see* Home
Nurturing, 26, 32, 42, 51, 52, 61

O

Object, 53–63, 69, 85–86, 88, 128
Oedipal, 58
Olney, James, 130
Online, 16, 64, 72
  See also Blog
Onlooker, 36, 37, 44, 60, 70, 72, 84, 85, 109, 111, 121, 123
  See also Eye contact; Viewer

P

Pain, 2, 14, 24, 32, 35, 38, 60, 63, 67, 87, 88, 91, 93
Painting, 107–109
  See also Drawing; Picture book
Parent
  parental, parenthood, 19, 65, 67
  parent-child inversion, parent as patient, parent-turned-patient, 20, 41, 46
Parkinson's disease, 18, 78, 92–93
  See also Dementia; Lewy body dementia
Partial View, 11, 83–86
  See also Henderson, Cary Smith

Partner, partnership, 19, 37–39, 57, 72, 83, 110, 120, 129
  See also Couple; Husband; Spouse; Wife
Past
  vs. future, 8, 100–101
  vs. present, 31, 53, 56, 65, 67, 71–72, 79, 87, 100–101, 127
Pathography, 6, 24, 103
  See also Account
Patient
  experience, 6, 9, 12, 20, 26, 79
  identity, 9, 20, 40–46, 82, 110
Pearl, *see* Images
Performance, *vs.* description of disease, 11, 84, 89
  See also Basting, Anne Davis
Personhood, 8, 38, 62, 72, 76, 78, 82, 86, 97, 101, 110, 130
Pharmaceutical care, 17, 59, 65, 105
Phenomenology, 130
Philosophy, 10, 41, 56
Phoenix, *see* Images
Photo
  photo book, 16, 36–38, 45, 58–65
  photograph (close-up), 31, 42, 52, 58, 63, 85, 106, 111, 123, 127
  photographing, 25, 31, 36–37
  portrait, 58, 60, 61
Photographer, 26, 36–37, 52, 59, 60, 85, 111
Physician, 92
  See also Clinician; Doctor
Picture book, 16, 33–35, 123
  See also Drawing; Painting
Placement, *see* Home
Plot, 14, 21, 78
Poetics, 6, 11, 13–14, 42, 56, 73, 94, 98, 130
Poetry, 38, 119
Policy, 6, 25, 51, 77, 99, 130, 132

Politics, 4, 6, 11–13, 17, 21, 40, 78, 91–94, 98, 102, 118, 120, 123, 125, 127–132
Postmodern, 89–90, 103–110, 115, 116
Preconceptions, 21, 46, 58, 100, 122, 128
Present, *see* Past
Print-on-demand, *see* Book
Professional, *see* Caregiver
Prominent, celebrity patient, 93, 113–115
    See also Famous
Prophet, patient as postmodern, 103–110
Psychoanalytical, 10, 58, 60, 130
Publisher, 16, 17, 43, 83, 101, 106, 108, 113, 114
Puzzle. Journal d'une Alzheimer, 107–110
    See also Couturier, Claude

R
Rabins, Peter V., 34
Race, 15, 19
Readership, 17, 78, 91, 108
Reagan, Nancy Davis, 13
Rebirth, *see* Images
Recognition, 12, 61–62, 71, 126, 128
Reliability, 13, 73
Religion
    Buddhist, 44
    Christian, 79–81, 104
    God, 80, 107, 112
    See also Faith; Spirituality
Respect, 31, 51, 110, 112
Retrospective, 39, 105, 108
River, *see* Images
Roach, Marion, 50, 68
Rohra, Helga, 98, 110–113, 115, 116, 118, 127

Rose, Larry, 76–78, 80, 82–83, 100, 102–103, 106, 109
Rota, Nucci A., 30, 51

S
Sabat, Steven R., 2, 6, 63, 86
Scarry, Elaine, 38, 87
Scar Tissue, 24–25
    See also Ignatieff, Michael
Schneider, Charles, 81, 103, 109
Self-help, 113, 115
Selfhood, 9, 11, 12, 61
Shadow, *see* Images
Shell, *see* Images
Shenk, David, 41
Ship, *see* Images
Show Me the Way to Go Home, 79
    See also Rose, Larry
Sieveking, David, 51, 119, 123–127
Silence, 38–43, 53, 70, 99
Smith, Sidonie, 13, 32
Social
    social constructionist, 10, 21, 89
    sociocultural, 5, 6, 46, 128, 132
    socio-economic, 12, 15, 19, 22, 96, 98, 132
    sociopolitical, 4, 92, 96, 123
Son, 20, 51, 55–68, 86, 112, 124, 127
Sontag, Susan, 14, 85
Spain, Spanish, 4, 15, 123, 125
Speechlessness, 37, 87, 102, 122
Spirituality, spiritual, 10, 81, 100, 103
    See also Faith; God; Religion
Spohr, Betty Baker, 26, 33–35, 37–38, 40–42, 44–45, 51, 69, 80, 85, 87, 105, 107
Spouse, 18, 25, 26, 33–40, 51, 69, 115, 128
    See also Couple; Husband; Partner; Wife

Stages, *see* Alzheimer's Disease; Dementia
Stigma, 4, 6, 12, 46, 62
Storyline, 31, 91, 96, 127
Strange Relation, 38–40, 129
   See also Hadas, Rachel
Strawson, Galen, 55–56
Stress, 42, 128
   See also Care – burden
Stroke, 18, 33, 43
   See also Transient ischemic attack
Subjectivity, 8, 76, 102
Suicide, *see* Assisted suicide
Surprise, 43, 105, 106
Survival, survivor, as in triumphalist narratives, 7, 32, 42, 67, 92, 94, 104, 106, 113

T

Tangles, 119–123
   See also Leavitt, Sarah
Tape recording, 84, 98
Taylor, Richard, 97, 101–103, 105, 114–116, 118
Teaching, training, 17, 26, 40, 42–43, 59, 61, 64, 67, 105, 116, 127, 132
Toledano, Phillip, 52, 62–64, 68, 84, 86, 100, 109, 111, 118, 123
Torture, *see* Images
Transient ischemic attacks (TIA), 18, 31
   See also Stroke
Trebus project, 71
Triumphalist narrative, 7, 32, 91–93
   See also Survival
Truth, narrative, 32, 56

U

United Kingdom, 3, 4
   See also Britain, British; England, English

United States, 4, 85
   See also America
Upbringing, 20, 46, 51–52, 68
   See also Education

V

Vascular dementia, 18, 55
Vegetable, *see* Images
Venturino, Giovanna, 29
Verdict, *see* Images
Vergiss Mein Nicht, 123–127
   See also Sieveking, David
Vickers, Neil, 130
Victim, *see* Images
Viewer, 61, 63, 70–72, 111, 123, 126
   See also Onlooker
Voyeurism, 37
Vulnerability, 4, 36, 52, 91

W

Wall, Frank, 51, 104
War, 65, 70, 86–87
Watson, Julia, 13, 32
Weakness, 91, 119, 124
Wellbeing, 52, 69, 100, 107, 110
Western, 6, 15, 17, 76, 85, 90, 131
   See also America; Austria; Canada; Europe; France; Germany; Italy; Spain; United Kingdom; United States
Wheelchair, 2, 59, 70–72
Whitehouse, Peter J., 88
Who Will I Be When I Die?, 76, 104
   See also Boden, Christine
Wife, 33–40, 51, 55, 57, 61, 63–64, 83–85, 93, 108, 124, 126, 127
   See also Couple; Partner; Spouse
Wilhoit, Mary, 28, 64
Williams, Ian, 121

Wilson, A. N., 55
Wiltshire, John, 12, 24–25, 76–77, 129, 131
Wisdom, 52, 65
Woodward, Kathleen, 25, 50–51, 68, 96, 131

Z
Zabbia, Kim Howes, 109
Zacharias, Sylvia, 57–58, 98
Zeilig, Hannah, 4, 132
Zimmermann, Christian, 96, 100, 111, 118

The manufacturer's authorised representative in the EU is Springer Nature Customer Service Centre GmbH, Europaplatz 3, 69115 Heidelberg, Germany. If you have any concerns regarding our products, please contact ProductSafety@springernature.com

Printed and bound by CPI Group (UK) Ltd, Croydon, CR0 4YY

23/03/2026

02076402-0011